The Anti-Inflammatory Diet
Slow Cooker Cookbook

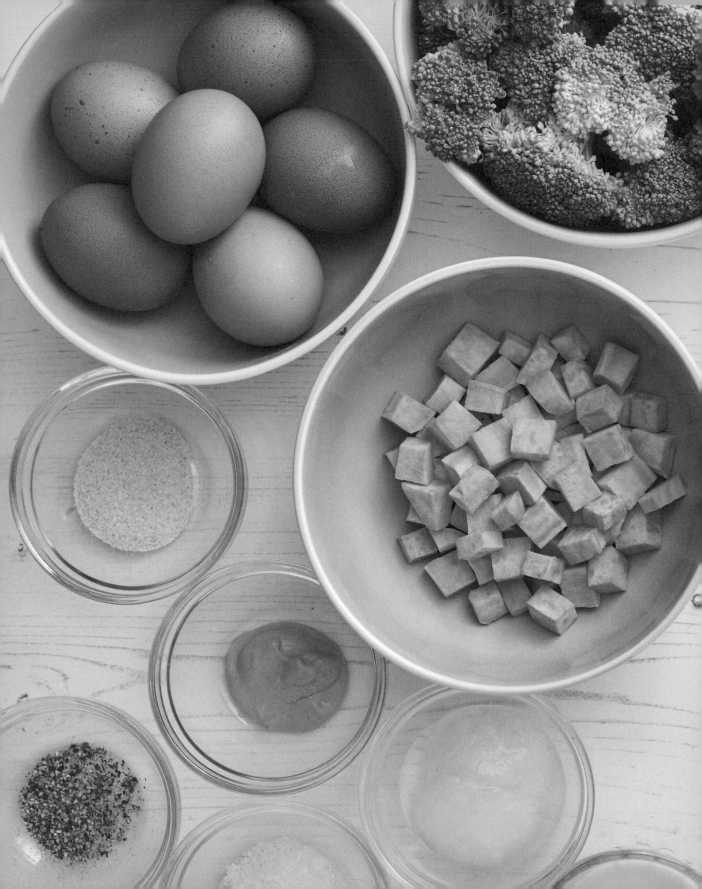

THE Anti-Inflammatory Diet

SLOW COOKER COOKBOOK

PREP-AND-GO RECIPES FOR LONG-TERM HEALING

MADELINE GIVEN, NC

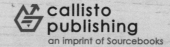

callisto
publishing
an imprint of Sourcebooks

Published by Callisto Publishing LLC C/O Sourcebooks LLC

P.O. Box 4410, Naperville, Illinois 60567-4410

(630) 961-3900

callistopublishing.com

Printed and bound in the United States of America.

VP 16

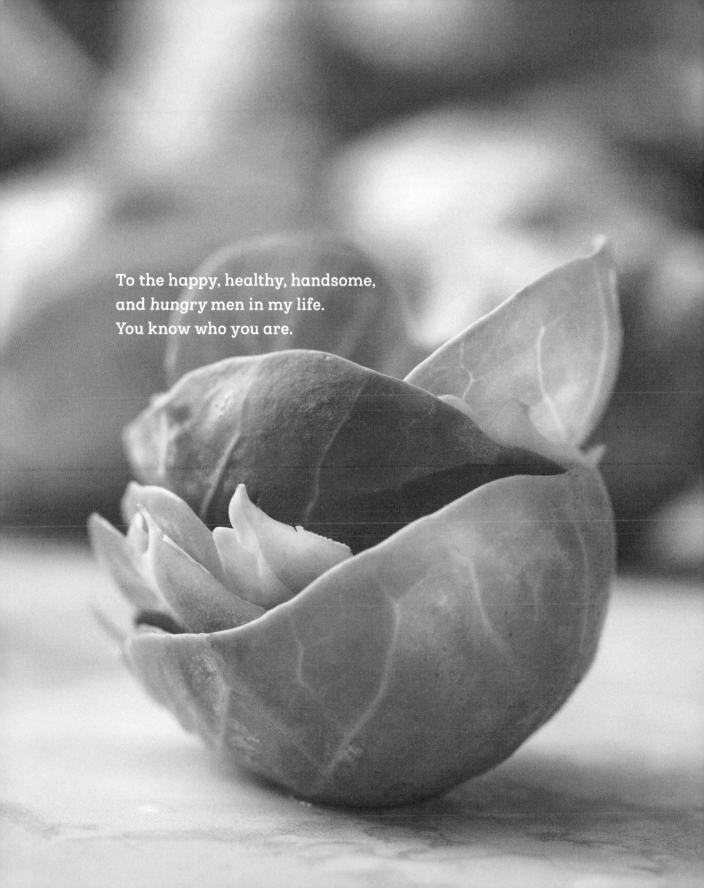

To the happy, healthy, handsome,
and hungry men in my life.
You know who you are.

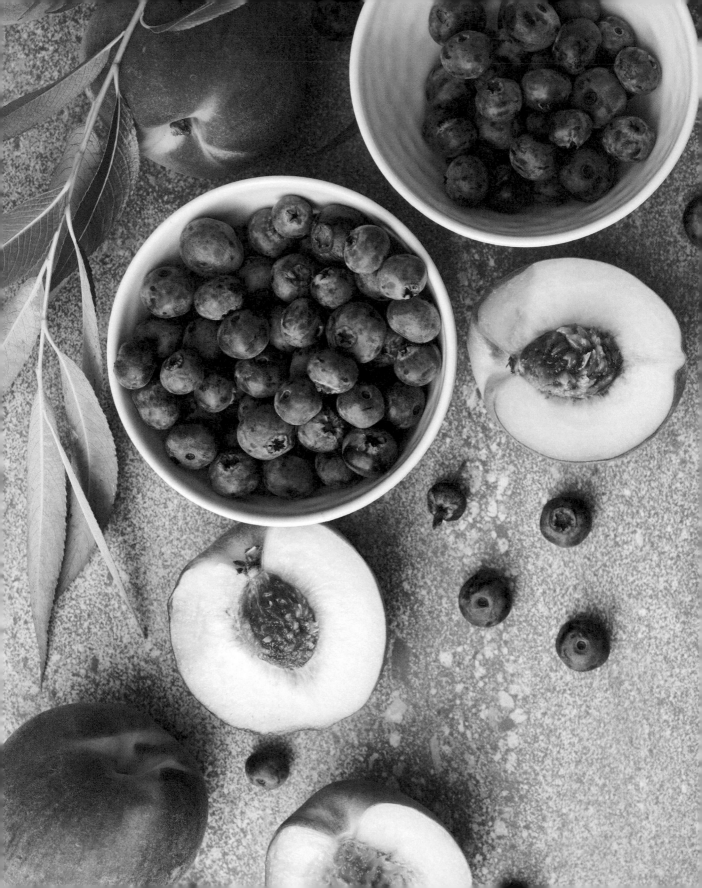

Contents

4 | Plant-Based Mains   43

5 | Poultry   67

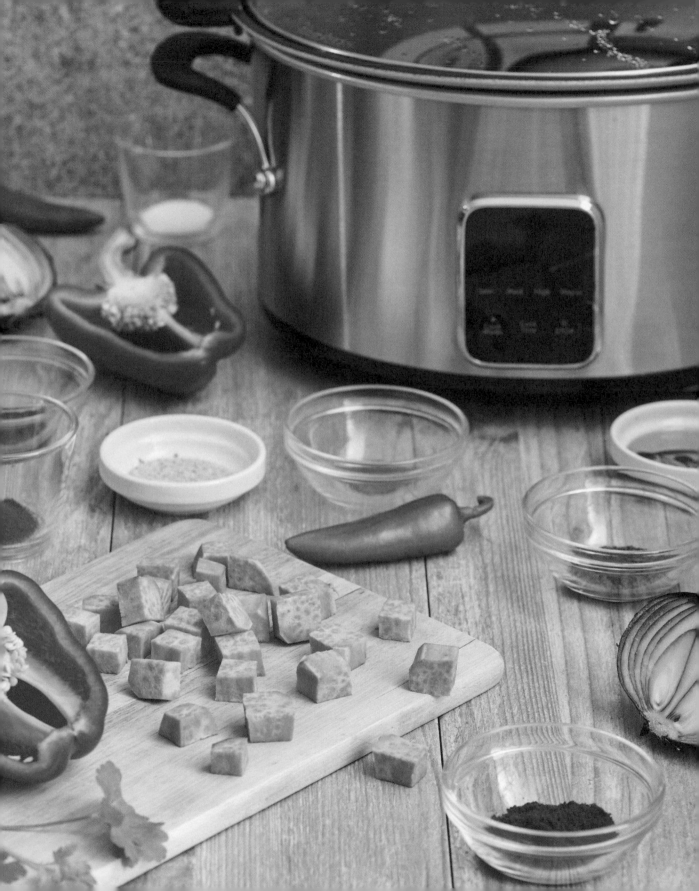

Introduction

IF YOU'VE PICKED UP THIS BOOK, inflammation must be on your mind—fighting it, preventing it, and staying healthy every day. You've come to the right cookbook! I'll teach you how to fight inflammation using recipes with minimal prep work and simple ingredients. They also taste amazing so you won't get bored. And using a slow cooker to make them means it does most of the work. Even the act of cooking foods for longer periods using lower heat can be beneficial to your health. Fewer nutrients are destroyed in the process, and more of the fats remain stable and unbroken. This means you receive more of the energy food has to give you, without the inflammatory damage it can so often do through rancid oils and fried elements.

I used to associate slow cookers with grandmothers, unhealthy casseroles, and greasy bakes. Now I know better! The slow cooker has proved itself time and again to be a miracle gadget that cooks in a slow and healthy way as long as you put ingredients into it that help, not harm, your body. Relying on my slow cooker has made a huge difference in making the most of my time and energy, ensuring my family eats well.

As a new mom, who is also a nutritionist, my days fill up fast...faster than I ever thought possible...and things such as self-care can end up taking a backseat. For me, self-care includes good nutrition and making healthy meals. I'm sure your days are just as busy, and, let's face it, the last thing anyone needs at the end of a chaotic day is the added stress of wondering what to make for dinner—a simple question turned dreaded dilemma. This is where I can help. With a little humility and some hard-earned wisdom, I've managed to make creating fresh and healthy meals part of my daily multitasking—but not without a lot of help from the slow cooker.

I can't help but think of clients I worked with over the years to create meal plans that included tasty and healthy recipes to manage their inflammation.

Some of these clients included busy parents with young children at the top of their priority lists. Being single at the time, though, I couldn't fully realize there was far too much prep work, long ingredient lists, and too much time required for grocery shopping—not to mention the actual cooking. I'm in awe of how they managed it all—including staying healthy and inflammation free—but I also know now there is a simpler way. My new approach to everyday meal prep is inspired by them.

My goal in writing these recipes is to prove that embarking on a new-to-you diet doesn't have to be full of restrictions to get the results you need. With a little background knowledge and the proper guidebook (this cookbook!), you'll be able to focus on the joy of the incredibly lush and flavorful, inflammation-busting ingredients you *do* get to eat. Chances are, you will never notice the lack of gluten, dairy, soy, sugar, or a host of other inflammation-causing ingredients—and you'll feel much better in the process.

Get ready to add a little dinner anticipation to your morning routine. By merely tossing a bit of goodness into your slow cooker and flipping a switch before you start your day, you'll be welcomed home at dinnertime by inviting aromas rather than the stress of daunting meal prep—or worse, inflammation-inducing takeout. And the same goes for breakfast. While you sleep, you'll rest easy knowing that when you wake up, your slow cooker will offer up a nourishing meal to power you through the day.

One versatile kitchen appliance, less inflammation, and a happier, healthier life.

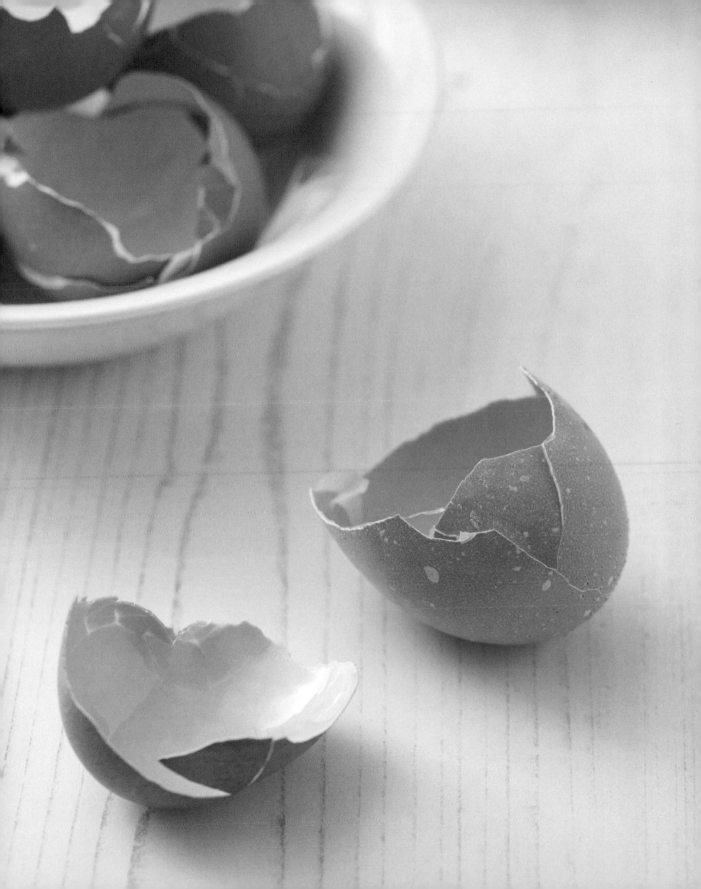

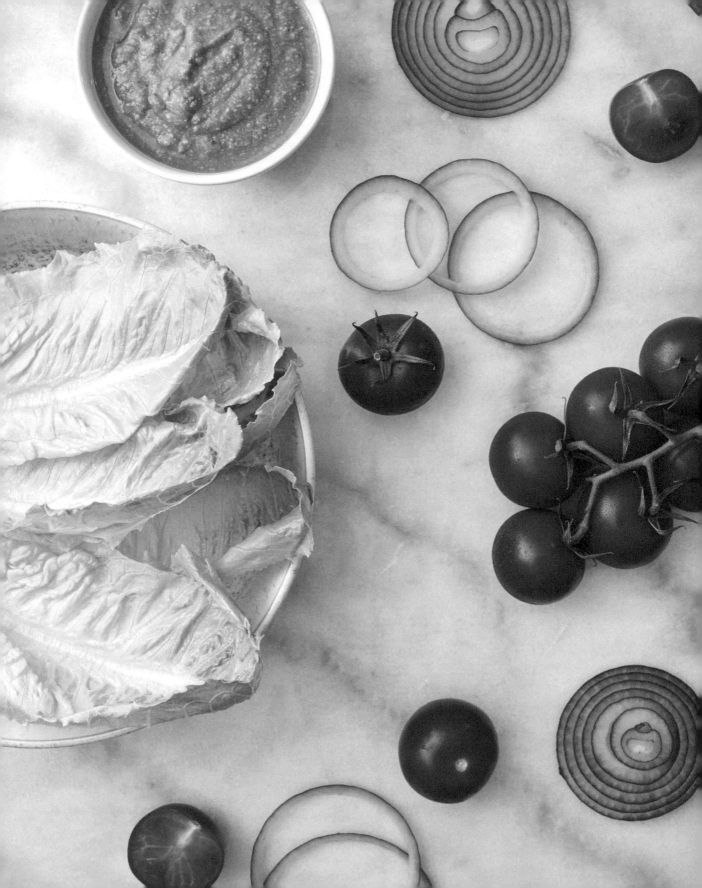

1 | Slow Cooking on the Anti-Inflammatory Diet

If you're looking to follow a more anti-inflammatory diet—whether short term to manage symptoms or long term to help maintain a healthy eating plan—the slow cooker takes the extra hands-on prep time out of the equation and makes cooking with real-food ingredients approachable for all. You'll quickly find how easy it is to counter our fast-food culture effectively by promoting the slow-food movement in your own home with the ease of a single pot. Many slow cooker recipes are even colloquially referred to as "dump recipes" because they allow you to, literally, dump ingredients into a single pot and leave it for up to eight hours, when you can then return to a warm, ready-to-eat meal.

Basic Principles of the Anti-Inflammatory Diet

To grasp the basic principles of inflammation, picture a fire. Acute inflammation is beneficial to the body because it cleanses the body of disease and starts the healing process, much like a well-contained wildfire that clears off old brush and disease.

On the other side of the spectrum, *chronic* inflammation is better compared to a never-ending, damp, smoldering fire. If left unaddressed in the body, it will result in an ever-increasing number of immune cells fighting an endless battle at the inflammation site, leading to serious disease.

Think of *acute* inflammation as fast acting, high level, and healing, whereas chronic inflammation is lingering, low level, and self-perpetuating.

WHOLE GRAINS

This is your chance to eat whole grains, prepared the old-fashioned way. Whole grains—grains that haven't been milled, refined, or stripped of their natural nutrients—retain their original fiber content, meaning they help promote a healthy digestive tract. Because whole grains take longer to digest than refined grains, they work to keep your blood sugar under control by improving insulin sensitivity. They also keep you feeling fuller longer so your appetite stays in check. The slow cooker really lends itself beautifully to whole grains, such as quinoa, brown rice, and ancient grains, and their desire to cook long and slow.

EAT THE ORGANIC RAINBOW

When you consume a colorful rainbow of organic fruits and vegetables, you're feeding your body with foods known for their phytonutrients, which fight inflammation in the body and provide a wealth of antioxidants to ward off oxidative stress caused by free radicals. This, essentially, means fighting degenerative disease in the body (which is caused by the oxidation). Berries are some of the fruits lowest on the glycemic index, so they minimally affect your blood sugar, and most research is in agreement that sugar intake is the main culprit of many diseases, including cardiovascular disease, type 2 diabetes, fatty liver, leaky gut, and more. Dark leafy greens contain both vitamin K and omega-3 fatty acids—big players in the fight against inflammation in the body. Some studies even suggest vitamin K destroys inflammatory cells that contribute to rheumatoid arthritis (RA). By slow cooking these more delicate ingredients over low heat, fewer nutrients will be broken down or lost in the process, allowing your body to reap even greater benefits from these foods.

FLAVORFUL HERBS AND SPICES

Include herbs and spices in every dish. Spices such as cinnamon, garlic, ginger, and turmeric are powerful inflammation fighters, and can also make flavorful additions to a meal any time of day. Each has its own unique health properties. For example, cinnamon helps regulate blood sugar; unregulated blood sugar can lead to insulin resistance and/or type 2 diabetes. Insulin can then affect bodily tissues and increase stored fat, which produces chemicals that lead to more inflammation. Garlic contains sulfur, which encourages the immune system to fight disease, and turmeric contains curcumin, which modifies immune system responses, stopping inflammation in its tracks. Slow cooking with these aromatic ingredients means variety and flavor in every inflammation-fighting bite. We will also be using sea salt, as opposed to table salt, because it is typically less refined and maintains its original mineral content.

HEALTHY FATS

Don't fear fat! While certain fats (such as trans fats) have a well-deserved bad rep, there are many fats that actually protect against inflammation in the blood vessels, such as the fatty acids found in flaxseed. Avocados contain phytosterols with inflammation-blocking properties. And unadulterated olive oil contains high levels of monounsaturated fats to protect a healthy heart from inflammation. Many of these fresh fats can be drizzled or layered onto your completed meal once it's out of the heat zone in the slow cooker for even more inflammation-regulating goodness on your plate.

FOOD SENSITIVITIES AND ALLERGIES

Pay attention to your body and its reaction to different foods. Food intolerances can completely disrupt your digestive tract while also stirring up inflammation in the rest of the body as well. If you're merely sensitive to a food, it will mainly bother your gut, whereas a true allergy can cause reactions throughout your entire immune system within seconds of consuming it. The recipes I've developed for you here specifically omit some of the most common reactionary foods, such as gluten, dairy, and soy, so you don't need to worry about adjusting them to suit your goals.

A HEALTHY GUT

Heal your gut from the start. It's the body's main defense against invaders that can cause inflammation. When embarking on a new health trajectory, it's important to set yourself up for success as much as possible. Change is hard, but by focusing at the start on healing from the inside out, you'll do yourself a huge favor, and inflammation will begin to calm before you know it.

Consuming plenty of probiotic-rich and fermented foods helps rebuild and feed your gut's microbiome. The gut microbiome consists of a community of bacteria that live inside our digestive tracts, doing a plethora of tasks including fighting off intruding bacteria and helping break down our food; thus, they are important when it comes to immunity/wellness and keeping inflammation in check. Recipes such as Coconut-Vanilla Yogurt (page 107) contain live and active cultures to repopulate the good bacteria in your body, while comforting bone broths (pages 68 and 86) contain soothing amino acids such as l-glutamine that heal the lining of your digestive tract.

The overall effect of eating foods such as these, while a complicated process, is simply to help bring our digestive tracts (and ultimately, our whole bodies) back toward their original, whole, untainted, and fully healthy states. This occurs through healing of the mucosal gut lining, repopulation of the good bacteria in the microbiome, and soothing any inflammation present in the digestive tract.

Foods that Fight Inflammation

Try to think of anti-inflammatory eating as an act of empowerment! You've been given the chance to heal your own body. The following points prove that the choices of anti-inflammatory foods far outweigh any restrictions, so there's no need to begin with trepidation—eating through the recipes in this book may be more enjoyable than you previously thought!

FISH

The most widely sought omega-3 fatty acids are found in wild-caught oily fish such as salmon. Just because you won't find many seafood recipes in this slow cooker cookbook (their delicate nature doesn't hold up well under such long cooking times) doesn't mean you shouldn't monitor your daily omega-3 intake! If you feel that fish are too pesky to prepare or expensive to purchase, try a supplement with krill or cod liver oil to increase these inflammation-fighting fats in your body. Fish also contain vitamin D. Insufficient vitamin D is associated with many inflammatory disease states.

DARK LEAFY GREENS

Dark green leafy vegetables contain ample amounts of vitamin K, an antioxidant known for reducing inflammatory markers in the body. Toss handfuls of fresh kale, cabbage, and spinach into recipes to add more of this essential nutrient to your diet.

FRESH HERBS

Culinary herbs are so versatile: They increase flavor, aroma, and the healing power of a meal all with one sprinkle or dash. Start with more familiar herbs such as basil, oregano, and rosemary. Basil contains compounds called eugenols that rival over-the-counter anti-inflammatory drugs. Explore other herbs and spices to keep things interesting, too.

PREBIOTICS

Prebiotic fibers are indigestible plant fibers that make their way to the large intestine and feed the probiotic bacteria living there. Common foods such as raw onion, asparagus, and banana contain noteworthy amounts of prebiotic fiber to encourage a healthy gut.

PHYTONUTRIENTS

Phytonutrients are essentially beneficial plant chemicals occurring naturally in colorful fruits and veggies. They are believed to fight disease in the body. The decrease in inflammation brought on by consuming fiber-rich fruits and vegetables may actually have more to do with these special substances than the fiber element itself. Eat up!

FRUIT ENZYMES

Tropical fruits, such as pineapples and papayas, contain naturally occurring enzymes called papain and bromelain. These proteolytic enzymes (enzymes in our bodies that specifically break down proteins, as opposed to fats or carbs) help your body digest certain tough food compounds more efficiently, lowering overall inflammation in the gut. You can also buy these digestive enzymes in supplement form from your local health store.

The Foods that Worsen Inflammation

Picture the following foods as if they were waving big red flags, because they all promote inflammation in the body. Become as familiar as you can with them so you can easily avoid purchasing them at the grocery store, or worse—eating them! If some of your favorite foods fall into this list, you may find you stop craving them if you intentionally and completely avoid them for a couple of weeks.

REFINED CARBOHYDRATES

Refined carbohydrates include things such as white flours, sugars, pasta, and breads, which have all been stripped of their precious fiber and nutrients, resulting in a far more negative impact on your blood sugar. In turn, these sugary foods fuel the production of advanced glycation end products (AGEs) that stimulate inflammation.

SEAFOOD AND THE SLOW COOKER

Daily fish consumption is highly beneficial when our bodies are fighting inflammation. Seafood contains high levels of the highly favored omega-3 fatty acids, which decrease the production of pro-inflammatory compounds in the body. Wild-caught seafood is ideal, but many sustainable farming practices are popping up around the world as well. If you live near the ocean, check out a local fishermans' market for the freshest possible fish (and nutrients!).

Unfortunately, for our purposes here (slow cooking), seafood doesn't fare well in the slow cooker. The longer cooking times are not ideal for their delicate layers. Thankfully, there are numerous amazingly simple ways to prepare tasty fish dishes without the use of the trusty slow cooker. I encourage you to think outside the box (or the slow cooker!) and creatively find ways to get more wild-caught seafood into your diet. To help with this, I've included a guide for cooking four popular seafood entrées, along with the slow cooker recipes from this book that they'll pair best with. Enjoy!

Salmon

To make simple and tasty salmon, in a small bowl, stir together 1 teaspoon each of garlic powder, dried basil, and salt. Sprinkle it evenly on top of four servings of salmon (usually about 2 to 3 ounces each). In a cast iron skillet over medium heat, heat 1 tablespoon of avocado oil. Add the salmon and cook for about 5 minutes per side, until it begins to flake. Remove it from the heat and let rest for at least 5 minutes before serving with lemon wedges for squeezing.

Suggested pairings: Mediterranean Quinoa with Peperoncini (page 37) or Herbed Harvest Rice (page 39).

Shrimp

Coat 1½ pounds shrimp in equal parts lemon juice and olive oil (about 2 tablespoons each) and sprinkle with 1 teaspoon each of salt and garlic powder. Heat a grill pan (or outdoor grill) to medium-high heat. Place the shrimp in the pan (or on the grill) and cook for 2 to 3 minutes per side, until opaque.

Suggested pairings: Coconutty Brown Rice (page 38) or Cauliflower "Rice" Risotto (page 48).

Mussels

In a large pot over high heat, combine 1 tablespoon of olive oil with 1 teaspoon each of dried basil and garlic powder. Add 1 cup broth of your choice to the pot and a large splash of white wine. Once boiling, add 4 pounds of mussels (scrubbed and debearded) to the pot. Cover the pot and cook for 5 minutes. Open the lid and give it a few good stirs before re-covering the pot and cooking for about 5 more minutes, or until the mussels have opened. Discard any that do not open.

Suggested pairings: White Bean & French Onion Soup (page 54) or Sweet Potato & Leek Soup (page 51).

Cod

Preheat the oven to 425°F. Drizzle 4 cod fillets with 2 tablespoons lemon juice and ½ teaspoon each sea salt and freshly ground black pepper. Cut four pieces of parchment paper about four times the size of each fillet. Place each fillet in the center of a piece of parchment, and drizzle with olive oil. Close each packet by sealing and crinkling the paper into a pouch. Place the pouches on a baking sheet and bake for about 25 minutes, or until the fish flakes easily with a fork.

Suggested pairings: Balsamic Beets (page 62) or Maple-Dijon Brussels Sprouts (page 61).

By consuming simple sugars such as the ones just listed, your body runs the risk of becoming insulin resistant and setting off a cascade of issues with the way it processes sugars. This can lead to a host of diseases, such as those mentioned previously, all of which include inflammation that specifically affects some part of the body. Because these types of ingredients are more often found in fast-food and takeout restaurants, it's best to avoid these easy, yet dangerous, food alternatives altogether.

TRANS FATS

Trans fats and rancid oils (when a fat oxygenates and begins to deteriorate) are big no-nos on the anti-inflammatory diet. Thankfully it's easy to avoid overheating fats in a slow cooker, since the temperatures are kept on the low side. And because we're eating whole foods here, trans fats are naturally eliminated from our plates.

ALLERGENS

If you know you're allergic to a particular food, don't eat it. Logical, right? But what if you don't know? One of the main symptoms of an allergic reaction to a food is inflammation, even if you can't see or feel it. So it may be a good idea to be tested for food allergies and be knowledgeable about your body. That way, you can consciously avoid all foods that trigger an inflammatory response. Common allergens include wheat gluten, dairy, peanuts, corn, soy, and eggs.

DAIRY

Commercial dairy is a different food than fresh-from-the-cow dairy. Commercial dairy is most often homogenized, pasteurized, and preserved with chemicals. It's devoid of the natural enzymes that help your digestive tract properly break down its proteins. For those still wanting some dairy in their lives, but without the associated symptoms, raw milk from a trusted source or cultured dairy such as yogurt or kefir can be excellent options.

GLUTEN

Gluten has been a hot-button word for more than a decade, and it mostly lives up to its hype. It's a simple protein in wheat that acts like glue, making bread delicious. Unfortunately, that glue can also muck up our insides due to how extremely difficult it is to properly digest. Whenever our bodies have to work harder to perform a simple task such as digestion, especially with a tricky protein like gluten, irritation can occur, resulting in internal inflammation and all its associated symptoms.

SOY

Soy has a lengthy rap sheet in the world of nutrition. Much of the soy in the United States has been genetically modified, which by itself has caused widespread allergies and digestive upset. It also contains phytic acid, which is an indigestible anti-nutrient that can actually prevent our bodies from properly absorbing other nutrients. And last but not least, the phytoestrogens naturally found in soy have been linked to autoimmune disease and cancer.

If you tend to eat a lot of soy because you purposely avoid meat in your diet, I usually recommend simply omitting those meat products and not replacing them with "fake meat products." For example, veggie sausage is typically made of mostly vital wheat gluten and soy proteins and is highly processed. You can, however, rely on other forms of natural, vegetarian protein, such as other legumes (black or pinto beans, for example), nut butters, quinoa, and eggs, all of which are included in recipes throughout this book.

SETTING UP YOUR ANTI-INFLAMMATORY SLOW COOKER KITCHEN

Using less electricity than an oven, a slow cooker has the ability to beautifully tenderize even the toughest cuts (and happily, the most inexpensive cuts) of meat without the added grease or preservatives you find in fast food. By cooking foods slowly at lower temperatures, you extract maximum flavor from ingredients, sans the common inflammation culprits such as gluten, dairy, and overheated and rancid fats. Your meals cook in their own juices or sauces rather than added fat, and they retain more of their natural vitamin and mineral content than fried or boiled foods. And, while cooking this way does take more time, it all happens while you are away doing something else. It's like having a personal chef on staff!

Bear with me as I wax scientific for a moment. I briefly mentioned *advanced glycation end products*, or AGEs, earlier. These compounds are produced most often when sugars combine with specific amino acids or fats in a process called *glycation*. When AGEs accumulate in your body, they majorly contribute to chronic inflammation. Sounds scary, but here's an important tip to help avoid taking on any more AGEs in your body: More AGEs form when foods such as meat are cooked using dry-heat methods at high temperatures (grilling, searing, frying, etc.).

Steaming and stewing—similar to what goes on under the lid of a slow cooker—are methods that help the foods retain moisture at lower temperatures, decreasing the risk of adding more AGEs to your diet. Big win, and you'll feel better for it.

SUPER (SLOW COOKER) FOODS

Like most kitchen appliances, there are certain foods that lend themselves to specific cooking processes, and other foods that don't. Let's quickly discuss some healthy, inflammation-lowering ingredients that will make the most of your slow cooker's energy.

PANTRY ESSENTIALS

Alliums: Garlic and onions not only add depth of flavor to virtually any meal but also suppress inflammatory markers in the body. Both keep for weeks in the pantry, so they're easy to have on hand.

Beans: These inexpensive, long-cooking pantry staples are high in fiber and extremely versatile. Be sure to soak them overnight first and dump the water before cooking—they'll be far easier to digest!

Coconut oil: The lauric acid in coconut oil contains anti-inflammatory properties, making it a great fat choice.

Dried spices and herbs: Many of my recipes call for dried or powdered spices and herbs because they are simply easier to keep on hand. Fresh is best, but high-quality pantry spices are great in a pinch! If you do use fresh herbs, multiply the amount of dried herbs called for in the recipe by three for the right quantity.

Nuts and nut butters: Some nuts and seeds are high in alpha linoleic acid, which is a type of anti-inflammatory omega-3 fatty acid. Almonds and walnuts are good to keep on hand.

Oats: Choosing carbohydrates that take longer to digest, such as oats, means fewer blood sugar spikes, which can be very beneficial in reducing inflammation.

Olive oil: The phenolic compounds in olive oil (there are 36!) have many powerful anti-inflammatory properties—one is even said to work as well as ibuprofen!

Quinoa: Quinoa is often mistaken for a grain, but it is actually a seed. (You'll still find it in the Beans & Grains chapter here, because it functions much like a grain in meals.) It packs an inflammation-fighting punch with its high fiber and protein content, but, similar to beans, it's very important to soak it overnight before cooking and consuming because it contains a protective indigestible layer that is damaging to the human gut.

Root vegetables: Deeply colored root vegetables, such as powerful purple beets and oh-so-good orange sweet potatoes, contain many anti-oxidant flavonoids, which are highly anti-inflammatory.

REFRIGERATOR ESSENTIALS

Bone broths: Using your slow cooker, it's easy to make your own Chicken Bone Broth (page 68) or Beef Bone Broth (page 86) with recipes in this cookbook. If buying from the store, however, purchase a trusted, slow-cooked brand. If I don't make my own, I like RoliRoti Butcher's Bone Broth; Epic brand, Bonafide Provisions, and Kettle & Fire.

Cruciferous vegetables: This potent anti-inflammatory vegetable family, which includes broccoli and cauliflower, has a positive effect on the biological factors that stir up inflammation in the body. Choose broccoli, kale, or cauliflower to hold up well in a slow cooker.

Dark leafy greens: You'll be amazed how easy it is to sneak a handful of healthy greens, such as spinach or kale, into many recipes and watch them wilt away, barely noticeable to potentially picky eaters. But the benefits remain.

Eggs, pastured and organic: You'll notice a big difference in freshness, taste, and that beautiful deep, bright orange yolk when you purchase high-quality eggs. Healthier chickens mean healthier eggs for you.

Flaxseed: They're tiny, but these seeds are an excellent plant-based source of omega-3 fatty acids. They keep best when refrigerated, especially if they've already been ground.

Frozen organic vegetables: This one is a bit of a trick because you'll read in the next few pages you should never put frozen food in a slow cooker because it messes dangerously with the temperature. However, it's not always possible to have fresh vegetables stocking your fridge, so having precut frozen vegetables on hand means you can thaw them the night before you need them and save money and time in the process—and still eat your veggies!

Garlic: Hate chopping garlic? Then don't! Grab a jar of minced garlic and keep it in your fridge.

Pasture-raised meats: Cows raised 100 percent on grass produce beef higher in omega-3 fatty acids, the antioxidant vitamin E, and the plant pigment beta-carotene. Getting more omega-3s (instead of omega-6s) and the other nutrients mentioned above into your diet is connected with less inflammation. And vice versa—beef not raised correctly is going to have more chemicals, antibiotics, hormones, and pro-inflammatory compounds such as omega-6s, which ultimately wreak havoc in many of the body's systems, causing joint pain, heart disease, fatty liver disease, and more. Choose organic, free-range, and grass-fed meats and poultry whenever possible.

Squeeze-tube herbs: These little market finds are a quick way to cheat on your fresh herbs. You can find anything from cilantro to ginger in paste form that can sit in your fridge for weeks. Tomato paste comes in tubes now, as does anchovy paste—flavor in an instant.

ESSENTIAL EQUIPMENT

Cooking with a slow cooker doesn't require a lot of specialized equipment—other than the slow cooker—but a few essentials you may even already own will make the process that much easier, especially if you're dealing with the pain of inflammation. Here is what I recommend:

Electric can opener: Don't fight through the literal pain of trying to wind up a manual can opener. You'll love using an electric version that requires only quick contact, and . . . voilà!

Jar gripper: This little piece of silicone can make you suddenly feel like you have Popeye strength when it comes to really tough stuck jar lids.

Immersion blender: It's often quicker to use an immersion blender to cream soups and mash cooked beans, so it's handy to have one of these also.

High-speed blender: Sometimes it's too much work to use an immersion blender to cream soups in the slow cooker. Invest in a high-speed blender to do the work for you. It will also come in handy for making smoothies that include anti-inflammatory super-foods and powders.

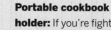

Portable cookbook holder: If you're fighting inflammation in your hands, flipping the pages of a book can bring a lot of pain. Using a cookbook holder eases the pain *and* the frustration of having to find your page repeatedly.

KNOW YOUR SLOW COOKER

When used correctly, a slow cooker can effectively replace a number of tools, appliances, and other kitchen items. You can downsize by getting rid of your rice cooker and any extra-large and hard-to-store pots. If you haven't already purchased a slow cooker, don't be overwhelmed by the many options! I break them all down here for you.

- Both round and oval slow cookers are available. Round ones tend to use less counter space while still offering the same volume. Oval slow cookers are more likely to fit an entire bird or certain kinds of roasts.

- A volume of 6 quarts is an average for popular modern slow cookers, and that's the size this cookbook uses most often. However, as long as yours is in the 5- to 7½-quart range, you should be fine. The majority of slow cookers available include low, high, and warm temperature settings. There are both manual and digital options, and each has its pros and cons. Manual cookers tend to cost less, while cookers with digital controls mean you can have your meal switched to warm when the cooking time is up, even if you're not home.

- As a general rule, although all brands differ some, the low setting on a slow cooker is about 190°F and the high setting is about 250°F. For the recipes in this book, we'll use the low setting most of the time so you have more time in between to focus on creating spaces for health and fun in your life. It's also worth noting that, for the most part, nutrients are damaged less at lower temperatures than at higher temperatures. Our goal is to preserve as many of those inflammation-fighting antioxidants as possible!

- Specially made slow cooker liners and bags are available to make cleanup even faster, but these are typically made from plastic. There is concern that chemicals from the liners can leach into food during the elongated cooking time. When food sticking may be an issue, I call for coating the cooker pot with a healthier alternative, such as olive or coconut oil.

SLOW COOKER DOS AND DON'TS

DO

- Be sure to cut heartier vegetables into similar-size pieces so they cook at the same rate.

- Set a timer that you're likely to have with you (such as one on your phone) so you don't forget about your meal waiting to welcome you home!

- Use wooden or silicone utensils when stirring, scraping, and cleaning the slow cooker to avoid scratching the glaze in the lining of your pot.

- Submerge your meats completely if you want them to tenderize to the point of falling apart.

- Cut any oversized vegetables or pieces of meat in half if they won't fit properly into your slow cooker.

DON'T

- Peek! Lifting the lid to look or stir (unless a recipe explicitly calls for it) allows precious heat to escape, disrupting the cooking temperature and drawing the cooking time out even longer. Some pots now have clear lids so you can "peek" without lifting that lid.

- Use frozen food unless the recipe specifically calls for it. The frigid ingredients will keep the whole meal at potentially unsafe temperatures (40°F to 140°F) for too long, putting the whole dish—and your diners—at risk for unsafe food.

- Attempt seafood. While fish can be a huge part of the anti-inflammatory diet—and you should definitely include it for its wonderful health benefits—there are simply better ways to cook seafood than with a slow cooker. I include some specific options for you on page 7. Fish becomes too delicate over the long haul of the slow cooker cooking time, while shellfish barely need any time at all to cook and therefore become rubbery when made in a slow cooker.

- Cook vegetables that are too fragile for the long cook time, such as tomatoes, eggplant, zucchini, and asparagus. Unless you're planning to blend them into a sauce, avoid using the slow cooker for these veggies because the long cook time leaves them mushy (and no one likes mushy vegetables).

- Add extra liquid the recipe doesn't call for. Because the slow cooker lid is kept on, tight, little to no evaporation will occur, so you do not need extra liquid. This is why most liquids used in the recipes in this book will be packed-with-flavor broths as opposed to plain water.

About the Recipes

Consuming foods prepared and cooked properly and thoroughly is one of the dietary keys to lowering inflammation in the body. Thankfully, the slow cooker does the grunt work for you, helping you easily stay on track.

I've planned recipes here specifically designed to help you fight inflammation, so you can feel better and live healthier. To that end, you'll find recipes with the following labels to help you easily decide which to choose, based on your tolerances. They are:

- Corn Free
- Dairy Free
- Egg Free

- Gluten Free
- Nightshade Free
- Nut Free

- Soy Free
- Sugar Free
- Vegan

Prep times and cook times are listed at the top of each recipe so you'll know just how many minutes to set aside in the morning, or evening, before starting your slow cooker. Rest assured, I've kept these as short as possible, and many small steps can be done the night before to help your morning run even smoother.

At the end of each recipe you'll find tips for making your slow cooking experience even more educational and easier at the same time. Make-ahead suggestions for faster prep and ingredient substitutions are designed to help you tailor recipes to your needs. All recipes also contain full nutrition information so you can make the best decisions for your health. We'll also let you in on the amount of macronutrients in each recipe (fats, proteins, and carbohydrates), as well as some of their many subsets, such as sugars, fiber, cholesterol, and saturated fat.

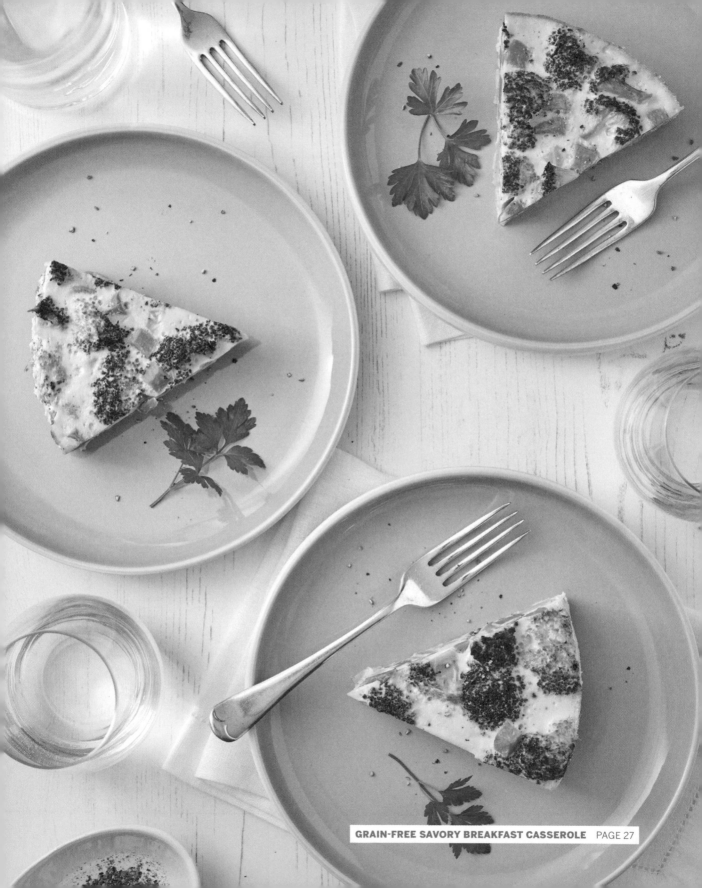

GRAIN-FREE SAVORY BREAKFAST CASSEROLE   PAGE 27

2 | BREAKFAST

Sweet Potato Home Fries

CORN FREE | DAIRY FREE | EGG FREE | GLUTEN FREE | NUT FREE | SOY FREE | SUGAR FREE | VEGAN

While the title is a bit of a misnomer because these aren't truly *fried*, the breakfast section on any menu isn't complete without proper home fries. This sweet potato version is no exception, and sweet potatoes are an excellent source of complex carbohydrates, vitamins B_6 and C, and dietary fiber. Working together, these antioxidants can reverse inflammation in the body. Add a dash of red pepper flakes if you want some kick.

SERVES 4 TO 6

Prep time: 15 minutes or fewer

Cook time: 6 to 8 hours on low

3 tablespoons extra-virgin olive oil, plus more for coating the slow cooker

2 pounds sweet potatoes, diced

1 red bell pepper, seeded and diced

½ medium onion, finely diced

1 teaspoon garlic powder

1 teaspoon sea salt

1 teaspoon dried rosemary, minced

½ teaspoon freshly ground black pepper

1. Coat the slow cooker with a thin layer of olive oil.

2. Put the sweet potatoes in the slow cooker, along with the red bell pepper and onion. Drizzle the olive oil as evenly as possible over the vegetables.

3. Sprinkle in the garlic powder, salt, rosemary, and pepper. Toss evenly to coat the sweet potatoes in the oil and seasonings.

4. Cover the cooker and set to low. Cook for 6 to 8 hours and serve.

PREPARATION TIP: Save some prep time while adding extra nutrition to this dish by keeping the sweet potato skins on. The skins contain a wealth of fiber and potassium. Just scrub and clean them well before dicing.

Serving Size: 4 servings

Per Serving: Calories: 296; Total Fat: 11g; Total Carbs: 48g; Sugar: 10g; Fiber: 7g; Protein: 4g; Sodium: 705mg

Perfect Hard-boiled Eggs

CORN FREE | DAIRY FREE | GLUTEN FREE | NIGHTSHADE FREE | NUT FREE | SOY FREE | SUGAR FREE

Eggs are high in omega-3 fatty acids. Interestingly, eggs from chickens fed a poor diet tend to have more omega-6 pro-inflammatory compounds, while eggs from chickens fed a flax meal–enriched diet have more omega-3s. Hard-boiled eggs make the perfect protein-rich, handheld breakfast, but they can be annoying to get right on the stove top. Adding vinegar to the cooking water greatly increases the ease with which they peel afterward.

SERVES 6

Prep time: 15 minutes or fewer
Cook time: 2½ hours on high

6 large eggs
1 tablespoon distilled white vinegar

1. Place the eggs along the bottom of the slow cooker, making sure none are stacked.

2. Add enough water to the slow cooker to just cover the eggs. Add the vinegar.

3. Cover the cooker and set to high. Cook for 2½ hours. Let cool before serving.

PREPARATION TIP: Gently place the eggs in a bowl of ice water as soon as the cook time is up to make them even easier to peel.

Serving Size: 1 egg
Per Serving: Calories: 74; Total Fat: 5g; Total Carbs: 1g; Sugar: 1g; Fiber: 0g; Protein: 6g; Sodium: 70mg

Chicken-Apple Breakfast Sausage

CORN FREE | DAIRY FREE | EGG FREE | GLUTEN FREE | NIGHTSHADE FREE | NUT FREE | SOY FREE | SUGAR FREE

Parsley is not the most common herb to have dried and on hand in your pantry. However, you can purchase inexpensive dried parsley flakes at the grocery store and use them as a powerful dose of green inflammation-fighting power in many savory recipes. They're full of plant flavonoids and have also been noted as a natural diuretic to help your body's detoxification processes.

SERVES 4 TO 6

Prep time: 15 minutes or fewer

Cook time: 6 to 8 hours on low

1 pound ground chicken

½ medium apple, peeled and minced

1 teaspoon sea salt

½ teaspoon freshly ground black pepper

½ teaspoon dried parsley flakes

½ teaspoon garlic powder

½ teaspoon dried basil leaves

¼ teaspoon ground cinnamon

1. In a large bowl, combine the chicken, apple, salt, pepper, parsley flakes, garlic powder, basil, and cinnamon. Mix well. Press the chicken mixture into the bottom of your slow cooker, ensuring it's a thin layer throughout.

2. Cover the cooker and set to low. Cook for 6 to 8 hours, or until the meat is completely cooked through.

3. Using a silicone spatula, loosen the chicken from around the edges and transfer to a cutting board. Cut into desired shapes (sticks or circles are common) and serve.

MAKE-AHEAD TIP: Make a full batch of these to freeze for later. Keep in an airtight container and, when you're ready to eat, heat the sausage (no need to thaw) in a skillet over medium-low heat for 8 to 10 minutes, turning often.

Serving Size: 4 servings

Per Serving: Calories: 210; Total Fat: 12g; Total Carbs: 4g; Sugar: 2g; Fiber: 1g; Protein: 21g; Sodium: 672mg

Golden Beet & Spinach Frittata

CORN FREE | DAIRY FREE | GLUTEN FREE | NIGHTSHADE FREE | SOY FREE | SUGAR FREE

This crustless quiche is an Italian favorite that's naturally free of refined flours. You can make this frittata your own by mixing and matching the vegetables you prefer, but use a combination of leafy greens and a heartier vegetable, such as broccoli, sweet potato, or bell pepper, that will withstand long, slow cooking.

SERVES 4 TO 6

Prep time: 15 minutes or fewer

Cook time: 5 to 7 hours on low

1 tablespoon extra-virgin olive oil

8 large eggs

1 cup packed fresh spinach leaves, chopped

1 cup diced peeled golden beets

½ medium onion, diced

¼ cup unsweetened almond milk

¾ teaspoon sea salt

½ teaspoon garlic powder

½ teaspoon dried basil leaves

Freshly ground black pepper

1. Coat the slow cooker with the olive oil.

2. In a large bowl, combine the eggs, spinach, beets, onion, almond milk, salt, garlic powder, and basil, and season with pepper. Whisk together and pour the custard into the slow cooker.

3. Cover the cooker and set to low. Cook for 5 to 7 hours, or until the eggs are completely set, and serve.

STORAGE TIP: This frittata should keep in the refrigerator for up to 3 days. Keep in mind that overheating the frittata to warm it could cause the eggs to become rubbery.

Serving Size: 4 servings
Per Serving: Calories: 202; Total Fat: 14g; Total Carbs: 6g; Sugar: 4g; Fiber: 1g, Protein: 13g; Sodium: 606mg

Sour Cherry & Pumpkin Seed Granola

CORN FREE | DAIRY FREE | EGG FREE | GLUTEN FREE | NIGHTSHADE FREE | SOY FREE | SUGAR FREE | VEGAN

The pumpkin seeds here are extremely high in antioxidants, and their omega-3 content has been shown to reduce arthritis-causing inflammation. Because it is virtually impossible to find store-bought granola devoid of inflammatory gluten and tons of added sugar, making your own is the solution. Thankfully it is a cinch, especially in a slow cooker. Another benefit to making your own is the freedom to add or remove ingredients to your liking—just keep the liquid to dry ingredients ratio the same.

SERVES 4 TO 6

Prep time: 10 minutes
Cook time: 5 to 6 hours on low

5 tablespoons melted coconut oil, divided

1 cup unsweetened shredded coconut

1 cup rolled oats

1 cup pecans

½ cup pumpkin seeds

1 ripe banana

1 tablespoon vanilla extract

½ teaspoon sea salt

½ teaspoon ground cinnamon

½ teaspoon ground ginger

1 cup dried sour cherries

1. Coat the slow cooker with 1 tablespoon of coconut oil.

2. In your slow cooker, toss together the coconut, oats, pecans, and pumpkin seeds.

3. In a small bowl, mash the banana with the remaining ¼ cup of melted coconut oil, the vanilla, salt, cinnamon, and ginger.

4. Add the liquid ingredients to the granola mixture and stir well to combine.

5. Cover the cooker and set to low. Cook for 5 to 6 hours (see Tip).

6. When the cooking is finished, stir in the cherries.

7. Spread the granola on a flat surface or baking sheet to cool and dry completely before storing in airtight containers. Stored in a cool place, this will keep up to six months.

IMPORTANT COOKING TIP: To get crispy granola, it's important that it loses its moisture in the cooking process. I usually don't recommend lifting the lid during the cook time, but in this case, you can leave the lid slightly ajar the entire cook time to vent condensation, or fit a dishtowel between the slow cooker and its lid to absorb condensation.

Serving Size: 4 servings
Per Serving: Calories: 777; Total Fat: 58g; Total Carbs: 58g; Sugar: 25g; Fiber: 10g; Protein: 7g; Sodium: 306mg

Morning Millet

CORN FREE | DAIRY FREE | EGG FREE | GLUTEN FREE | NIGHTSHADE FREE | NUT FREE | SOY FREE | SUGAR FREE | VEGAN

While millet is often referred to as a grain, it's technically an ancient grass seed with a similar structure to wheat. However, it's devoid of the gluten protein that puts wheat high on the inflammatory list. It also has a healthy dose of fiber that is protective of your entire digestive tract. In this recipe, millet combines with blueberries, which have a high antioxidant content and are them particularly anti-inflammatory. Blueberries are considered to be a protective fruit, meaning they help protect the brain and body from disease and further oxidative damage. Good morning, indeed.

SERVES 4

Prep time: 15 minutes or fewer

Cook time: 7 to 8 hours on low

1 cup millet

2 cups water

2 cups full-fat coconut milk

½ teaspoon sea salt

½ teaspoon ground cinnamon

½ teaspoon ground ginger

¼ teaspoon vanilla extract

½ cup fresh blueberries

1. In your slow cooker, combine the millet, water, coconut milk, salt, cinnamon, ginger, and vanilla. Stir well.

2. Cover the cooker and set to low. Cook for 7 to 8 hours.

3. Stir in the blueberries to warm at the end and serve.

INGREDIENT TIP: Having trouble finding millet at your local grocery store? It has become more popular over the last decade, so they're likely to have it stocked somewhere, usually in the organic foods aisle, or in the bulk dry goods section, where it's sure to be cheaper as well!

Serving Size: 4 servings

Per Serving: Calories: 276; Total Fat: 22g; Total Carbs: 18g; Sugar: 3g; Fiber: 1g; Protein: 3g; Sodium: 323mg

Caramel-Apple Oats

CORN FREE | DAIRY FREE | EGG FREE | GLUTEN FREE | NIGHTSHADE FREE | SOY FREE | VEGAN

Aside from their high fiber content that aids in balancing blood sugar, oats also contain compounds called *avenanthramides* that seem to play a role in reducing inflammation. By layering the ingredients, you give the apples a chance to really caramelize their natural sugars against the heat of the slow cooker coming through the coconut oil.

SERVES 4

Prep time: 15 minutes or fewer
Cook time: 6 to 8 hours on low

1 tablespoon coconut oil

3 sweet apples, such as Fuji or Gala, peeled and sliced

2 tablespoons coconut sugar

¼ teaspoon sea salt

1 teaspoon ground ginger

1 teaspoon ground cinnamon

1 teaspoon vanilla extract

2 cups rolled oats

1 cup unsweetened applesauce

3 cups unsweetened almond milk

½ cup water

1. Coat the slow cooker with the coconut oil.

2. Layer the sliced apples along the bottom of the slow cooker so each piece is touching the bottom.

3. In this order, layer in the coconut sugar, salt, ginger, cinnamon, vanilla, oats, applesauce, almond milk, and water.

4. Cover the cooker and set to low. Cook for 6 to 8 hours and serve.

NUTRITION TIP: If you want to be extra kind to your digestive tract, soak the oats in water the night before, and rinse and strain them before using in this recipe. Their starch will break down, helping them digest more easily, and their phytic acid content will be greatly reduced. As phytic acid is indigestible by humans and, therefore, causes digestive disrupt, the less of it, the better!

Serving Size: 4 servings
Per Serving: Calories: 313; Total Fat: 9g; Total Carbs: 56g; Sugar: 24g; Fiber: 8g; Protein: 6g; Sodium: 274mg

Carrot & Fennel Quinoa Breakfast Casserole

CORN FREE | DAIRY FREE | GLUTEN FREE | NIGHTSHADE FREE | SOY FREE | SUGAR FREE

A fun fact about fennel is that this mildly licorice-scented plant is fantastic at relieving menstrual cramps because it contains natural anti-inflammatory and antispasmodic properties. Though it's related to both parsley and carrots, it is still considered an herb in most chef circles.

SERVES 4 TO 6

Prep time: 15 minutes or fewer
Cook time: 5 to 7 hours on low

6 large eggs

½ cup quinoa, rinsed well (see Tip)

1½ cups unsweetened almond milk

½ teaspoon sea salt

½ teaspoon garlic powder

¼ teaspoon dried oregano

Freshly ground black pepper

1 fennel bulb, finely sliced

3 medium carrots, diced

1 tablespoon extra-virgin olive oil

1. In a medium bowl, whisk the eggs.

2. Add the quinoa, almond milk, salt, garlic powder, and oregano, and season with pepper. Whisk well until all ingredients are combined.

3. Stir in the fennel and carrots.

4. Coat the slow cooker with the olive oil, and slowly pour in the egg mixture.

5. Cover the cooker and set to low. Cook for 5 to 7 hours and serve.

NUTRITION TIP: Always rinse quinoa well to remove any oddities. This also helps break down any saponins that need to be stripped away to avoid bitterness or digestive upset.

Serving Size: 4 servings
Per Serving: Calories: 265; Total Fat: 13g; Total Carbs: 23g; Sugar: 2g; Fiber: 5g; Protein: 14g; Sodium: 526mg

Simple Steel-Cut Oats

CORN FREE | DAIRY FREE | EGG FREE | GLUTEN FREE | NIGHTSHADE FREE | NUT FREE | SOY FREE | SUGAR FREE | VEGAN

There really isn't a heartier breakfast cereal than traditional steel-cut oats. They digest more slowly and are lower on the glycemic index than regular rolled or quick oats, and therefore affect blood sugar less negatively. In other words, steel-cut oats are less likely to cause blood sugar spikes, which can, over time, lead to inflammatory diseases such as obesity and type 2 diabetes. Naturally high in fiber, steel-cut oats have a chewy texture and nutty taste. They can be tweaked myriad ways to create your preferred flavor. Try apples and cinnamon, bananas and walnuts, or cherries and almonds.

SERVES 4 TO 6

Prep time: 15 minutes or fewer

Cook time: 6 to 8 hours on warm

1 tablespoon coconut oil

4 cups boiling water

½ teaspoon sea salt

1 cup steel-cut oats

1. Coat the slow cooker with the coconut oil.

2. In your slow cooker, combine the boiling water, salt, and oats.

3. Cover the cooker and set to warm (or low if there is no warm setting). Cook for 6 to 8 hours and serve.

CLEANUP TIP: I wouldn't typically recommend using the warm temperature setting on your slow cooker as a go-to cooking solution, but for steel-cut oats, it creates a better texture with less mess, as the oats will boil and leave hard-to-clean residue on the high setting. Just make sure the water you use is *boiling* when you add it in at the start.

Serving Size: 4 servings

Per Serving: Calories: 172; Total Fat: 6g; Total Carbs: 27g; Sugar: 0g; Fiber: 4g; Protein: 6g; Sodium: 291mg

Grain-Free Savory Breakfast Casserole

CORN FREE | DAIRY FREE | GLUTEN FREE | SOY FREE | SUGAR FREE

This hearty breakfast casserole covers all the bases while boasting of one of the most powerful anti-inflammatory ingredients available to us–broccoli! As a cruciferous vegetable, broccoli has been shown to decrease the risk of both heart disease and cancer. Broccoli also contains sulfur compounds, which have a strong research track record when it comes to fighting inflammation.

SERVES 4 TO 6

Prep time: 15 minutes or fewer
Cook time: 4 to 5 hours on low

1 tablespoon coconut oil

6 large eggs

½ cup unsweetened almond milk

1 teaspoon Dijon mustard

1 teaspoon sea salt

1 teaspoon garlic powder

Freshly ground black pepper

1 cup broccoli florets

½ medium onion, diced

1 small sweet potato, peeled and diced

1 cup diced Chicken-Apple Breakfast Sausage (page 20)

1. Coat the slow cooker with the coconut oil.

2. In a medium bowl, whisk the eggs, almond milk, mustard, salt, and garlic powder, then season with pepper.

3. Put the broccoli, onion, sweet potato, and sausage in the slow cooker, and pour the egg mixture on top.

4. Cover the cooker and set to low. Cook for 4 to 5 hours, until the eggs are set and the vegetables are tender, and serve.

SUBSTITUTION TIP: If almond milk doesn't suit you, try another nondairy alternative such as hemp milk, cashew milk, or oat milk—just make sure they aren't sweetened or flavored!

Serving Size: 4 servings
Per Serving: Calories: 250; Total Fat: 14g; Total Carbs: 14g; Sugar: 6g; Fiber: 2g; Protein: 16g; Sodium: 908mg

German Chocolate Cake Protein Oats

CORN FREE | DAIRY FREE | EGG FREE | GLUTEN FREE | NIGHTSHADE FREE | SOY FREE | SUGAR FREE

As delicious and comforting as classic oatmeal is, it isn't necessarily the most well balanced of meals. By weight, raw oats are almost 80 percent carbohydrate (which includes fiber). Cacao, the unsweetened base of chocolate, has been shown not only to improve inflammatory conditions in the body, but also to work in the brain to lift mood and lower stress levels. This recipe adds some extra protein (collagen) and fat (coconut milk) to round out this family favorite.

SERVES 4 TO 6

Prep time: 15 minutes or fewer

Cook time: 6 to 8 hours on low

1 tablespoon coconut oil

2 cups rolled oats

2½ cups water

2 cups full-fat coconut milk

¼ cup unsweetened cacao powder

2 tablespoons collagen peptides (see Tip)

¼ teaspoon sea salt

2 tablespoons pecans

2 tablespoons unsweetened shredded coconut

1. Coat the slow cooker with the coconut oil.

2. In your slow cooker, combine the oats, water, coconut milk, cacao powder, collagen peptides, and salt. Stir to combine.

3. Cover the cooker and set to low. Cook for 6 to 8 hours.

4. Sprinkle the pecans and coconut on top and serve.

INGREDIENT TIP: Collagen peptides are one of the purest protein powders available today. It's made from the bones, skin, and connective tissue of animals (typically cows) and has incredible digestibility, amino acid content, and benefits for skin, hair, nails, bones, and joints in humans. Bonus—it's tasteless and dissolves almost instantly in liquid!

Serving Size: 4 servings

Per Serving: Calories: 457; Total Fat: 33g; Total Carbs: 36g; Sugar: 3g; Fiber: 7g; Protein: 10g; Sodium: 191mg

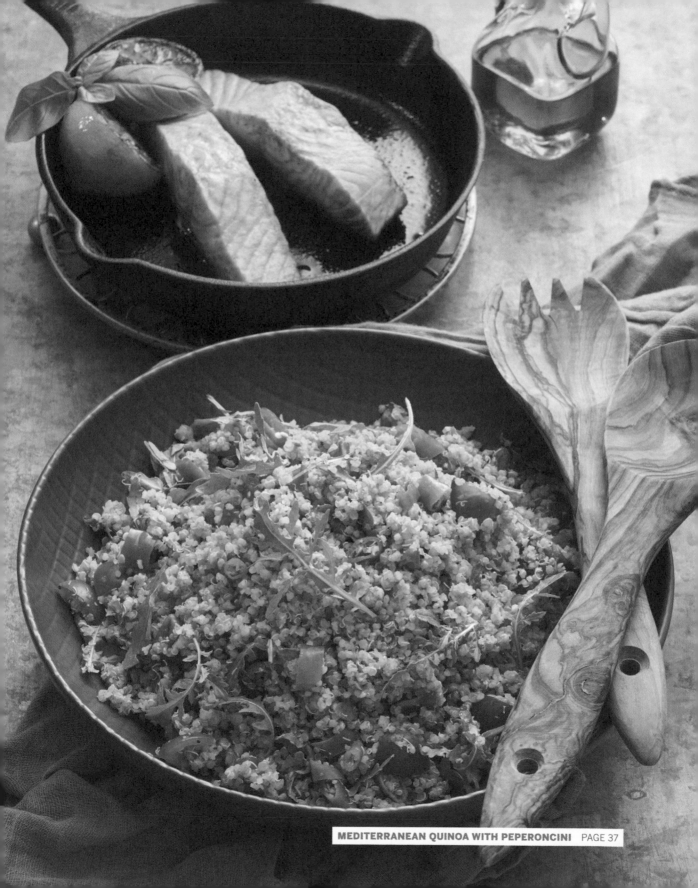

MEDITERRANEAN QUINOA WITH PEPERONCINI PAGE 37

3

BEANS & GRAINS

Basic Beans

CORN FREE | DAIRY FREE | EGG FREE | GLUTEN FREE | NIGHTSHADE FREE | NUT FREE | SOY FREE | SUGAR FREE | VEGAN

Beans of all shapes and sizes are known as the magical fruit, but what's the science behind all the noise? Beans contain sugars called *oligosaccharides* that go undigested in your digestive tract until they reach your colon, where they are readily digested by the bacteria that live there. The by-product of all this is, essentially, the gas that causes the flatulence so many people experience when consuming beans and legumes. However, this can be abated by using the method in this recipe. When you soak dried beans overnight in water, these sugars are lessened significantly. Just make sure you rinse them well before cooking! And the good news is, once you regularly have beans in your diet, your body will adjust and digest them with less fanfare.

MAKES 6 CUPS

Prep time: 8 hours to soak
Cook time: 7 to 8 hours on low

1 pound dried beans, any kind

Water

1. Rinse the beans, and pick out any broken ones or possible rocks or dirt particles.

2. Put the beans in a large bowl or in your slow cooker and cover with water. Let soak for a minimum of 8 hours, or overnight, at room temperature.

3. Drain and rinse the beans well. Put them in your slow cooker and cover with 2 inches of fresh water.

4. Cover the cooker and set to low. Cook for 7 to 8 hours, or until soft and cooked through. Drain and serve.

COOKING TIP: Add a strip of kombu seaweed to your cooking beans to help make them more digestible, especially if you don't have time to presoak. Kombu contains the enzymes needed to break down some of the oligosaccharides, called raffinose, in the beans. Look for it in the Asian foods section of your grocery store.

Serving Size: 1 cup
Per Serving: Calories: 259; Total Fat: 0g; Total Carbs: 48g; Sugar: 2g; Fiber: 19g; Protein: 15g; Sodium: 0mg

Vegan Baked Navy Beans

CORN FREE | DAIRY FREE | EGG FREE | GLUTEN FREE | NUT FREE | SOY FREE | VEGAN

Because beans are so high in fiber, they can lower inflammation simply by reducing the C-reactive protein levels in the body. These levels are a measure of inflammation in our bloodstreams. Most traditional baked bean recipes include bacon and a good amount of added sweeteners—no wonder they're so tasty! Here you'll find pure deliciousness, but without the processed sugars or meat. Be cognizant of choosing a ketchup and maple syrup that don't include high-fructose corn syrup or added fillers and preservatives.

SERVES 4 TO 6

Prep time: 15 minutes, plus 8 hours to soak

Cook time: 7 to 8 hours on low

2 cups dried navy beans, soaked in water overnight, drained, and rinsed (see Tip)

6 cups vegetable broth

¼ cup dried cranberries

1 medium sweet onion, diced

½ cup all-natural ketchup (choose the one with the lowest amount of sugar)

3 tablespoons extra-virgin olive oil

2 tablespoons maple syrup

2 tablespoons molasses

1 tablespoon apple cider vinegar

1 teaspoon Dijon mustard

1 teaspoon sea salt

½ teaspoon garlic powder

1. In your slow cooker, combine the beans, broth, cranberries, onion, ketchup, olive oil, maple syrup, molasses, vinegar, mustard, salt, and garlic powder.

2. Cover the cooker and set to low. Cook for 7 to 8 hours and serve.

COOKING TIP: It's extremely important to soak your beans before using them in a recipe. It reduces the phytic acid, reduces cooking time, ensures an even cooking experience, and allows your tummy the best (and least painful) experience as it digests them. You can even use the bowl of your slow cooker the night before to soak your beans in cool water with a dash of salt. Make sure it's at room temperature and the beans get at least an 8-hour bath. Rinse them well before using, and discard the soaking water.

Serving Size: 4 servings

Per Serving: Calories: 423; Total Fat: 11g; Total Carbs: 78g; Sugar: 25g; Fiber: 19g; Protein: 16g; Sodium: 1,731mg

Hatch Chile "Refried" Beans

CORN FREE | DAIRY FREE | EGG FREE | GLUTEN FREE | NUT FREE | SOY FREE | SUGAR FREE | VEGAN

Even though this recipe avoids frying, these cooked and mashed beans are as traditional as they come. The natural oils found in the cumin have been shown to contain compounds that block inflammatory pathways in the body. With the extra zest from the lime juice (feel free to add more!) and the flavor from the chiles and spices, you could also use this dish as a dip for bell pepper strips or chips.

SERVES 4 TO 6

Prep time: 15 minutes, plus 8 hours to soak

Cook time: 6 to 8 hours on low

2 cups dried pinto beans, soaked in water overnight, drained, and rinsed

7 cups vegetable broth

½ medium onion, minced

1 (4-ounce) can Hatch green chiles

1 tablespoon freshly squeezed lime juice

½ teaspoon ground cumin

½ teaspoon garlic powder

½ teaspoon sea salt

1. In your slow cooker, combine the beans, broth, onion, chiles, lime juice, cumin, garlic powder, and salt.

2. Cover the cooker and set to low. Cook for 6 to 8 hours, until the beans are soft.

3. Using an immersion blender, mash the beans to your desired consistency before serving. If you don't own an immersion blender, mash the beans by hand with a fork or a potato masher.

PREPARATION TIP: Instead of mincing the onion with a knife, you can get it even smaller by using a cheese grater and grating small bits of onion directly into the slow cooker.

Serving Size: 4 servings
Per Serving: Calories: 218; Total Fat: 0g; Total Carbs: 49g; Sugar: 6g; Fiber: 18g; Protein: 16g; Sodium: 1,287mg

Indian Butter Chickpeas

CORN FREE | DAIRY FREE | EGG FREE | GLUTEN FREE | SOY FREE | SUGAR FREE | VEGAN

This recipe is a bit of a play on words, as the traditional dish is actually butter *chicken*, hailing from the country of India. Loosely, it's a mild curry sauce, although there are many variations, with many different types of fat instead of butter. We're keeping it vegan and using a combination of coconut milk and a hint of almond butter to get that creamy finish with a lighter texture. The combination of the aromatic spices cumin, ginger, curry, and garlic give this recipe an inflammatory upper hand as they work together to aid in digestion and reduce inflammation.

SERVES 4 TO 6

Prep time: 15 minutes, plus 8 hours to soak

Cook time: 6 to 8 hours on low

1 tablespoon coconut oil

1 medium onion, diced

1 pound dried chickpeas, soaked in water overnight, drained, and rinsed

2 cups full-fat coconut milk

1 (14.5-ounce) can crushed tomatoes

2 tablespoons almond butter

2 tablespoons curry powder

1½ teaspoons garlic powder

1 teaspoon ground ginger

½ teaspoon sea salt

½ teaspoon ground cumin

½ teaspoon chili powder

1. Coat the slow cooker with coconut oil.

2. Layer the onion along the bottom of the slow cooker.

3. Add the chickpeas, coconut milk, tomatoes, almond butter, curry powder, garlic powder, ginger, salt, cumin, and chili powder. Gently stir to ensure the spices are mixed into the liquid.

4. Cover the cooker and set to low. Cook for 6 to 8 hours, until the chickpeas are soft, and serve.

SERVING TIP: For a complete meal, serve these over Coconully Brown Rice (page 38).

Serving Size: 4 servings

Per Serving: Calories: 720; Total Fat: 30g; Total Carbs: 86g; Sugar: 9g; Fiber: 19g; Protein: 27g; Sodium: 440mg

Basic Quinoa

CORN FREE | DAIRY FREE | EGG FREE | GLUTEN FREE | NIGHTSHADE FREE | NUT FREE | SOY FREE | SUGAR FREE | VEGAN

Keeping a container of cooked quinoa in your fridge for the week means you always have a creative base for quick or on-the-go meals in a pinch. It's an extremely versatile seed (although often treated as a grain) that is not only full of fiber but is considered a complete protein, as it has a full amino acid profile. Additionally, quinoa's fiber and protein help prevent blood sugar spikes that, over time, increase inflammation in the body through insulin resistance and ultimately can result in weight gain, diabetes, and a host of other life-threatening diseases.

SERVES 4 TO 6

Prep time: 15 minutes of fewer
Cook time: 4 to 6 hours on low

2 cups quinoa, rinsed well
4 cups vegetable broth

1. In your slow cooker, combine the quinoa and broth.

2. Cover the cooker and set to low. Cook for 4 to 6 hours. Fluff with a fork, cool, and serve.

STORAGE TIP: If you're making a large batch of quinoa to use for different salads and dishes throughout the week, don't add any dressings, sauces, or flavored liquids to it before refrigerating it or it will turn mushy. Keep the dressings and extras stored in separate containers until ready to eat, and then combine them.

Serving Size: 4 servings
Per Serving: Calories: 335; Total Fat: 5g; Total Carbs: 61g; Sugar: 2g; Fiber: 7g; Protein: 12g; Sodium: 550mg

Mediterranean Quinoa with Peperoncini

CORN FREE | DAIRY FREE | EGG FREE | GLUTEN FREE | NUT FREE | SOY FREE | SUGAR FREE | VEGAN

Here I'm making use of my favorite protein-rich seed that's often used as a grain (I've even included it in our Grains section!) because it comes out light and fluffy with a somewhat nutty flavor. The peperoncini, like all peppers, contain the compound capsaicin, which inhibits the inflammatory process by blocking specific pro-inflammatory compounds.

SERVES 4 TO 6

Prep time: 15 minutes or fewer
Cook time: 6 to 8 hours on low

1½ cups quinoa, rinsed well

3 cups vegetable broth

½ teaspoon sea salt

½ teaspoon garlic powder

¼ teaspoon dried oregano

¼ teaspoon dried basil leaves

Freshly ground black pepper

3 cups arugula

½ cup diced tomatoes

⅓ cup sliced peperoncini

¼ cup freshly squeezed lemon juice

3 tablespoons extra-virgin olive oil

1. In your slow cooker, combine the quinoa, broth, salt, garlic powder, oregano, and basil, and season with pepper.

2. Cover the cooker and set to low. Cook for 6 to 8 hours.

3. In a large bowl, toss together the arugula, tomatoes, peperoncini, lemon juice, and olive oil.

4. When the quinoa is done, add it to the arugula salad, mix well, and serve.

NUTRITION TIP: Adding leafy greens to warm dishes is a sneaky and excellent way to get in large portions of anti-inflammatory vegetables without the bulk or the taste, because they literally wilt to less than half their size compared to when they are consumed fresh.

Serving Size: 4 servings
Per Serving: Calories: 359; Total Fat: 14g; Total Carbs: 50g; Sugar: 2g; Fiber: 6g; Protein: 10g; Sodium: 789mg

Coconutty Brown Rice

CORN FREE | DAIRY FREE | EGG FREE | GLUTEN FREE | NIGHTSHADE FREE | NUT FREE | SOY FREE | SUGAR FREE | VEGAN,

Because brown rice still has its hull, it takes more time and more liquid to cook than white rice, which has been milled and refined to some degree. However, this also means that brown rice contains the natural fiber, vitamins, and minerals that white rice has been stripped of. Both brown and white rice can find their place in a nutrient-balanced diet, but I love the way the coconut milk soothes the tougher brown rice in this recipe.

SERVES 4 TO 6

Prep time: 15 minutes, plus
8 hours to soak

Cook time: 3 hours on high

2 cups brown rice, soaked
in water overnight, drained,
and rinsed

3 cups water

1½ cups full-fat coconut milk

1 teaspoon sea salt

½ teaspoon ground ginger

Freshly ground black pepper

1. In your slow cooker, combine the rice, water, coconut milk, salt, and ginger. Season with pepper and stir to incorporate the spices.

2. Cover the cooker and set to high. Cook for 3 hours and serve.

COOKING TIP: While it may be more convenient to use the low temperature setting for a longer cook time (ideally, while you're at work all day), brown rice doesn't do as well at the lower temperature, so using the high temperature for the time suggested is the best option here.

Serving Size: 4 servings
Per Serving: Calories: 479; Total Fat: 19g; Total Carbs: 73g; Sugar: 1g; Fiber: 4g; Protein: 9g; Sodium: 604mg

Herbed Harvest Rice

CORN FREE | DAIRY FREE | EGG FREE | GLUTEN FREE | NIGHTSHADE FREE | SOY FREE | VEGAN

Mushrooms have been shown to have a highly diverse molecular structure that includes many anti-inflammatory compounds. I suggest using cremini mushrooms for this recipe, although your favorite mushroom chopped small will work, too.

SERVES 4 TO 6

Prep time: 15 minutes, plus 8 hours to soak

Cook time: 3 hours on high

2 cups brown rice, soaked in water overnight, drained, and rinsed

½ small onion, chopped

4 cups vegetable broth

2 tablespoons extra-virgin olive oil

½ teaspoon dried thyme leaves

½ teaspoon garlic powder

½ cup cooked sliced mushrooms

½ cup dried cranberries

½ cup toasted pecans

1. In your slow cooker, combine the rice, onion, broth, olive oil, thyme, and garlic powder. Stir well.

2. Cover the cooker and set to high. Cook for 3 hours.

3. Stir in the mushrooms, cranberries, and pecans, and serve.

PREP TIP: Look for bags of frozen sliced mushrooms in the freezer section of your local grocery store, or buy presliced mushrooms and freeze them yourself, to save prep time. Just remember to stick them in the refrigerator the night before to thaw.

Serving Size: 4 servings

Per Serving: Calories: 546; Total Fat: 20g; Total Carbs: 88g; Sugar: 14g; Fiber: 7g; Protein: 10g; Sodium: 607mg

Spanish Rice

CORN FREE | DAIRY FREE | EGG FREE | GLUTEN FREE | NUT FREE | SOY FREE | SUGAR FREE | VEGAN

White rice isn't in and of itself inflammatory just because it's missing its outer hull. In fact, many nutritionists argue that because it has been stripped of that outer bran husk, it's actually easier to digest, and therefore causes even less inflammation in the gut.

SERVES 4 TO 6

Prep time: 15 minutes or fewer

Cook time: 5 to 6 hours on low

2 cups white rice

2 cups vegetable broth

2 tablespoons extra-virgin olive oil

1 (14.5-ounce) can crushed tomatoes

1 (4-ounce) can Hatch green chiles

½ medium onion, diced

1 teaspoon sea salt

½ teaspoon ground cumin

½ teaspoon garlic powder

½ teaspoon chili powder

½ teaspoon dried oregano

Freshly ground black pepper

1. In your slow cooker, combine the rice, broth, olive oil, tomatoes, chiles, onion, salt, cumin, garlic powder, chili powder, and oregano, and season with pepper.

2. Cover the cooker and set to low. Cook for 5 to 6 hours, fluff, and serve.

INGREDIENT TIP: When using canned tomatoes, look for those specifically marked as having a BPA-free lining.

Serving Size: 4 servings
Per Serving: Calories: 406; Total Fat: 7g; Total Carbs: 79g; Sugar: 5g; Fiber: 2g; Protein: 8g; Sodium: 1,058mg

Veggie "Fried" Quinoa

DAIRY FREE | EGG FREE | GLUTEN FREE | NIGHTSHADE FREE | NUT FREE | SOY FREE | SUGAR FREE | VEGAN

This is another quinoa recipe packed with fiber that helps produce a specific fatty acid that turns off genes related to inflammation and insulin resistance. It's a spin on traditional vegetable fried rice and is excellent topped with tamari, a gluten-free version of soy sauce. Or you can take it a healthy step further and use coconut aminos, a soy sauce substitute sans gluten *and* soy.

SERVES 4 TO 6

Prep time: 15 minutes or fewer

Cook time: 4 to 6 hours on low

2 cups quinoa, rinsed well

4 cups vegetable broth

¼ cup sliced carrots

¼ cup corn kernels

¼ cup green peas

¼ cup diced scallion

1 tablespoon sesame oil

1 teaspoon garlic powder

1 teaspoon sea salt

Dash red pepper flakes

1. In your slow cooker, combine the quinoa, broth, carrots, corn, peas, scallion, sesame oil, garlic powder, salt, and red pepper flakes.

2. Cover the cooker and set to low. Cook for 4 to 6 hours, fluff, and serve.

PREP TIP: Look for bags of frozen sliced vegetable combinations in the freezer section of your local grocery store to save prep time. Just remember to stick them in the refrigerator the night before to thaw.

Serving Size: 4 servings
Per Serving: Calories: 387; Total Fat: 8g; Total Carbs: 65g; Sugar: 4g; Fiber: 8g; Protein: 13g; Sodium: 1,147mg

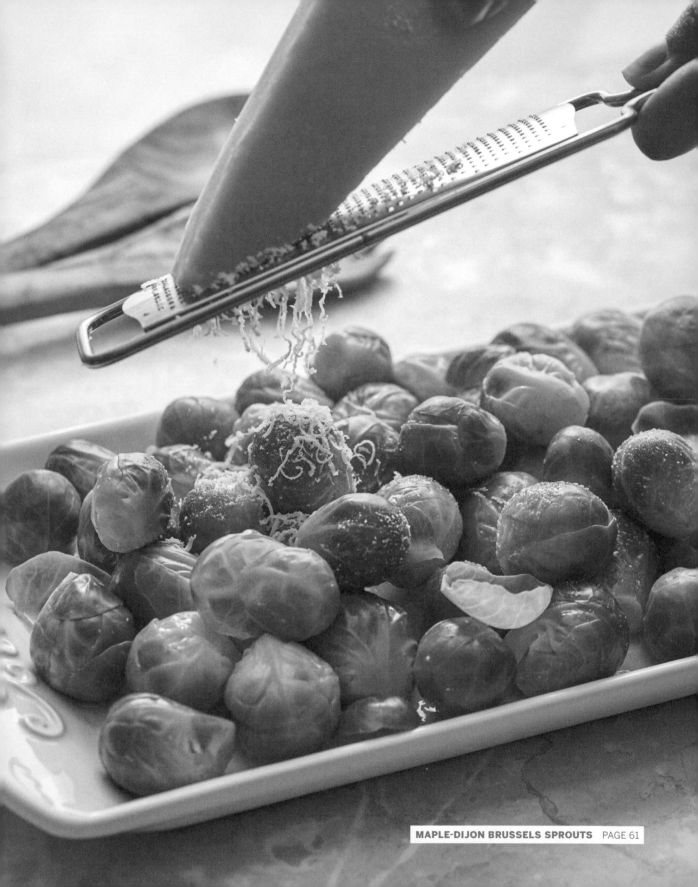

MAPLE-DIJON BRUSSELS SPROUTS PAGE 61

4 | PLANT-BASED MAINS

Classic Vegetable Broth

CORN FREE | DAIRY FREE | EGG FREE | GLUTEN FREE | NIGHTSHADE FREE | NUT FREE | SOY FREE | SUGAR FREE | VEGAN

Consuming vegetable broths is an amazing way to increase your daily intake of anti-oxidants, as the vitamins and minerals from the vegetable scraps leach into the liquid, leaving you with only the best inflammation-fighting broth around. By making your own vegetable broth, you are in complete control of the ingredients and can prevent any fillers, preservatives, or extra salt from being added. Some store-bought canned broths contain yeast extract, salt, flavoring, monosodium glutamate, caramel color, disodium guanylate, disodium inosinate, and soy lecithin. If that's not enough reason to make your own, I don't know what is!

MAKES ABOUT 12 CUPS

Prep time: 15 minutes or fewer
Cook time: 6 to 8 hours on low

Extra-virgin olive oil, for coating the slow cooker

6 cups veggie scraps (peels and pieces of carrots, celery, onions, garlic)

12 cups filtered water

½ medium onion, roughly chopped

2 garlic cloves, roughly chopped

1 parsley sprig

¾ teaspoon sea salt

½ teaspoon dried oregano

½ teaspoon dried basil leaves

2 bay leaves

1. Coat the slow cooker with a thin layer of olive oil.

2. In the slow cooker, combine the veggie scraps, water, onion, garlic, parsley, salt, oregano, basil, and bay leaves.

3. Cover the cooker and set to low. Cook for 6 to 8 hours.

4. Pour the broth through a fine-mesh sieve set over a large bowl, discarding the veggie scraps. Refrigerate the broth in airtight containers for up to 5 days, or freeze for up to 3 months.

INGREDIENT TIP: Don't use veggies from the Brassica family (broccoli, cabbage, etc.) because they unpleasantly affect the flavor.

Serving Size: 1 cup
Per Serving: Calories: 24; Total Fat: 0g; Total Carbs: 5g; Sugar: 2g; Fiber: 1g; Protein: 1g; Sodium: 202mg

Simple Spaghetti Squash

CORN FREE | DAIRY FREE | EGG FREE | GLUTEN FREE | NIGHTSHADE FREE | NUT FREE | SOY FREE | SUGAR FREE | VEGAN

Here's a spectacular way to make vegetables the main attraction, while also replacing a common ingredient that's typically full of gluten–spaghetti. Serve this spaghetti squash alongside Hearty Bolognese (page 89) or Pork Ragù (page 91), or with Garden Marinara Sauce (page 112).

SERVES 4 TO 6

Prep time: 15 minutes or fewer, plus 15 minutes to cool

Cook time: 8 hours on low

1 spaghetti squash, washed well

2 cups water

1. Using a fork, poke 10 to 15 holes all around the outside of the spaghetti squash. Put the squash and the water in your slow cooker.

2. Cover the cooker and set to low. Cook for 8 hours.

3. Transfer the squash from the slow cooker to a cutting board. Let sit for 15 minutes to cool.

4. Halve the squash lengthwise. Using a spoon, scrape the seeds out of the center of the squash. Then, using a fork, scrape at the flesh until it shreds into a spaghetti-like texture. Serve warm.

INGREDIENT TIP: When shopping for the perfect spaghetti squash, measure it to confirm it will fit into your slow cooker.

Serving Size: 4 servings
Per Serving: Calories: 60; Total Fat: 0g; Total Carbs: 15g; Sugar: 0g; Fiber: 0g; Protein: 0g; Sodium: 42mg

Stuffed Sweet Potatoes

CORN FREE | DAIRY FREE | EGG FREE | GLUTEN FREE | NUT FREE | SOY FREE | SUGAR FREE | VEGAN

The orange flesh of sweet potatoes is a source of antioxidant-rich nutrients, complex carbohydrates, vitamins B_6 and C, and beta-carotene, while the skin is high in dietary fiber. Working together, these elements can reverse inflammation in the body. I love choosing sweet potatoes over regular white potatoes because they are just plain good, and good for you. The best part is, no more dried-out baked potatoes—your slow cooker produces the moistest baked sweet potatoes you've ever tasted!

SERVES 4

Prep time: 15 minutes or fewer
Cook time: 6 to 7 hours on low

4 medium sweet potatoes

1 cup Hatch Chile "Refried" Beans (page 34)

4 tablespoons chopped scallions (both white and green parts)

1 avocado, peeled, pitted, and quartered

1. Wash the sweet potatoes, but do not dry them. The water left on the skins from washing is the only moisture needed for cooking. Put the damp sweet potatoes in your slow cooker.

2. Cover the cooker and set to low. Cook for 6 to 7 hours. A fork should easily poke through when they are done.

3. Carefully remove the hot sweet potatoes from the slow cooker. Slice each one lengthwise about halfway through. Mash the revealed flesh with a fork, and fill the opening with ¼ cup of beans. Top each with 1 tablespoon of scallions and a quarter of the avocado and serve.

SUBSTITUTION TIP: This is an extremely versatile recipe, as it allows you to stuff and top the sweet potatoes with your favorite ingredient combos. Here, I've created more of a Mexican-style dish, but you can try chopped red onion, cucumbers, and tomato to make it Greek, or be creative in the moment based on what's on hand.

Serving Size: 4 servings
Per Serving: Calories: 237; Total Fat: 8g; Total Carbs: 38g; Sugar: 7g; Fiber: 10g; Protein: 6g; Sodium: 315mg

Jam-Packed Peppers

CORN FREE | DAIRY FREE | EGG FREE | GLUTEN FREE | NUT FREE | SOY FREE | SUGAR FREE | VEGAN

Bell peppers are rich in several natural acids that have a strong anti-inflammatory effect on the body. Stuffed bell peppers are a visually impressive dish, but, using the slow cooker, the hands-on time is negligible and you can have a hearty, nutritious dinner on the table with one scoop. Choose bell peppers of any color, but remember that green tend to be the most bitter, then orange and yellow, with red being the sweetest of all.

SERVES 4

Prep time: 15 minutes or fewer

Cook time: 4 to 5 hours on low

1 tablespoon avocado oil

4 bell peppers, any color, washed, tops cut off, and seeded

½ cup water

2 cups Spanish Rice (page 40)

1 (15-ounce) can black beans, rinsed and drained well

1. Coat the bottom of the slow cooker with the avocado oil.

2. Place the peppers, upright, in the cooker. Add the water to the bottom of the slow cooker, around the outside of the peppers.

3. In a large bowl, stir together the rice and black beans. Stuff each pepper with one-quarter of the mixture.

4. Cover the cooker and set to low. Cook for 4 to 5 hours and serve.

COOKING TIP: Choose peppers that are roughly the same size and shape so they cook evenly and fit properly into your slow cooker. Cut a thin slice from the bottoms of the peppers if they are uneven and won't stand properly in your cooker.

Serving Size: 4 servings
Per Serving: Calories: 340; Total Fat: 9g; Total Carbs: 58g; Sugar: 3g; Fiber: 7g; Protein: 9g; Sodium: 687mg

Cauliflower "Rice" Risotto

CORN FREE | DAIRY FREE | EGG FREE | GLUTEN FREE | NIGHTSHADE FREE | NUT FREE | SOY FREE | SUGAR FREE | VEGAN

Forget the orange—cauliflower has 77 percent of your daily vitamin C requirement, which is a powerful, inflammation-fighting antioxidant we can all use more of. With just a few minutes of prep, you can turn this humble vegetable into a perfect substitute for rice. And what could be better use of rice than the Italian classic, risotto? Enjoy this "rice" dish alongside Beef & Bell Peppers (page 87) or Herbed Meatballs (page 90).

SERVES 4 TO 6

Prep time: 15 minutes or fewer

Cook time: 4 to 5 hours on low

1 pound riced cauliflower

1 celery stalk, minced

1 small shallot, minced

¼ cup vegetable broth

½ teaspoon garlic powder

½ teaspoon sea salt

Freshly ground black pepper

1. In your slow cooker, combine the riced cauliflower, celery, shallot, broth, garlic powder, and salt, and season with pepper. Stir well.

2. Cover the cooker and set to low. Cook for 4 to 5 hours and serve.

INGREDIENT TIP: Many grocery stores now carry riced cauliflower in their produce or freezer sections. If you can't find any, grate a head of raw cauliflower on a cheese grater, or roughly chop the entire head and place it in a food processor, pulsing lightly with the chopping blade until the desired consistency is reached.

Serving Size: 4 servings

Per Serving: Calories: 50; Total Fat: 2g; Total Carbs: 6g; Sugar: 2g; Fiber: 2g; Protein: 1g; Sodium: 888mg

Mushroom Risotto with Spring Peas

CORN FREE | DAIRY FREE | EGG FREE | GLUTEN FREE | NIGHTSHADE FREE | NUT FREE | SOY FREE | SUGAR FREE | VEGAN

True risotto can take hours of constant stirring and watching, but with this recipe, the slow cooker does all the cooking and tending for you. Porcini mushrooms add a wealth of protein that most risotto dishes otherwise lack, along with an incredible depth of flavor. Mushrooms are also believed to contain potent anti-inflammatory properties that reduce symptoms from diseases brought on by inflammatory conditions.

SERVES 4 TO 6

Prep time: 15 minutes or fewer

Cook time: 2 to 3 hours on high

1½ cups Arborio rice

1 cup English peas

1 small shallot, minced

¼ cup dried porcini mushrooms

4½ cups broth of choice (choose vegetable to keep it vegan)

1 tablespoon freshly squeezed lemon juice

½ teaspoon garlic powder

½ teaspoon sea salt

1. In your slow cooker, combine the rice, peas, shallot, mushrooms, broth, lemon juice, garlic powder, and salt. Stir to mix well.

2. Cover the cooker and set to high. Cook for 2 to 3 hours and serve.

TIME-SAVING TIP: Don't worry about rehydrating the dried mushrooms before cooking. The extra liquid in the recipe and slow cooking provide all the moisture and time they need to plump.

Serving Size: 4 servings

Per Serving: Calories: 382; Total Fat: 1g; Total Carbs: 79g; Sugar: 4g; Fiber: 3g; Protein: 12g; Sodium: 934mg

Split Pea & Carrot Soup

CORN FREE | DAIRY FREE | EGG FREE | GLUTEN FREE | NIGHTSHADE FREE | NUT FREE | SOY FREE | SUGAR FREE | VEGAN

Split peas are legumes that contain a wealth of protein and fiber, which means less room in their nutrient makeup for carbohydrates, which can raise the glycemic load of a food and spike blood sugar, causing inflammation in the body. This warming soup, with loads of nostalgia in every bite, has plenty of hardiness to make it perfect for freezing. The carrots take the place of the traditional ham here, while also adding their own subtle, sweet flavor. Split pea soup often thickens when stored, so stir in some extra vegetable broth before serving to thin it. For added umami without the meat, check out the tip.

SERVES 4 TO 6

Prep time: 15 minutes, plus 8 hours to soak

Cook time: 7 to 8 hours on low

2 cups dried split peas, soaked in water overnight, drained, and rinsed well

3 carrots, chopped

1 celery stalk, diced

½ medium onion, diced

1 tablespoon extra-virgin olive oil

1 tablespoon freshly squeezed lemon juice

2 teaspoons dried thyme leaves

1 teaspoon garlic powder

½ teaspoon dried oregano

2 bay leaves

8 cups broth of choice (choose vegetable to keep it vegan)

1. In your slow cooker, combine the split peas, carrots, celery, onion, olive oil, lemon juice, thyme, garlic powder, oregano, bay leaves, and broth.

2. Cover the cooker and set to low. Cook for 7 to 8 hours.

3. Remove and discard the bay leaves. For a smoother soup, blend with an immersion blender and serve.

INGREDIENT TIP: For an extra punch of flavor at the end, add 1 teaspoon of coconut aminos. If you're not sensitive to soy, add 1 teaspoon of tamari or miso paste (both are made from fermented soy).

Serving Size: 4 servings

Per Serving: Calories: 306; Total Fat: 4g; Total Carbs: 66g; Sugar: 9g; Fiber: 26g; Protein: 23g; Sodium: 1,156mg

Sweet Potato & Leek Soup

CORN FREE | DAIRY FREE | EGG FREE | GLUTEN FREE | NIGHTSHADE FREE | NUT FREE | SOY FREE | SUGAR FREE | VEGAN

I've snuck a bit of the anti-inflammatory spice turmeric into this classic soup recipe. Its bright yellow color blends in seamlessly with the sweet potatoes. Cumin is another spice with powerful health benefits—mostly in calming the digestive system. These spices blend well to complement the vegetables in this classic comfort soup. Drizzle a little olive oil on top before serving, if desired.

SERVES 4 TO 6

Prep time: 15 minutes or fewer

Cook time: 4 to 5 hours on low

5 medium sweet potatoes, peeled and chopped

1 leek, washed and sliced (see Tip)

1½ teaspoons garlic powder

1 teaspoon sea salt

½ teaspoon ground turmeric

¼ teaspoon ground cumin

4 cups vegetable broth

Freshly ground black pepper

1. In your slow cooker, combine the sweet potatoes, leek, garlic powder, salt, turmeric, cumin, and broth, and season with pepper.

2. Cover the cooker and set to low. Cook for 4 to 5 hours.

3. Using an immersion blender, purée the soup until smooth and serve.

PREP TIP: To wash a leek properly, cut it lengthwise once before slicing it crosswise. Fill a medium bowl with water and immerse all the chopped pieces into the water, swishing them around briskly. The dirt should sink to the bottom of the bowl while the leek pieces will float.

Serving Size: 4 servings

Per Serving: Calories: 200; Total Fat: 1g; Total Carbs: 46g; Sugar: 10g; Fiber: 6g; Protein: 3g; Sodium: 1137mg

Minestrone Soup

CORN FREE | DAIRY FREE | EGG FREE | GLUTEN FREE | NUT FREE | SOY FREE | SUGAR FREE | VEGAN

Classic minestrone soup hails from Italy and is typically made thick and packed with vegetables. It often includes rice or pasta. I've omitted the grains and gluten in this recipe, but, if it suits you, add some brown rice pasta.

SERVES 4 TO 6

Prep time: 15 minutes or fewer

Cook time: 6 to 8 hours on low

1 (14-ounce) can diced tomatoes with their juice

1 (14-ounce) can kidney beans, drained and rinsed well

2 celery stalks, diced

2 carrots, diced

1 zucchini, diced

1 small onion, diced

1 tablespoon freshly squeezed lemon juice

1 teaspoon sea salt

½ teaspoon garlic powder

½ teaspoon dried oregano

½ teaspoon dried basil leaves

½ teaspoon dried rosemary

2 bay leaves

6 cups vegetable broth

1 cup packed fresh spinach

1. In your slow cooker, combine the tomatoes, kidney beans, celery, carrots, zucchini, onion, lemon juice, salt, garlic powder, oregano, basil, rosemary, bay leaves, and broth.

2. Cover the cooker and set to low. Cook for 6 to 8 hours.

3. Remove and discard the bay leaves. Stir in the spinach and let wilt (about 5 minutes) before serving.

SUBSTITUTION TIP: Have you made your own slow cooker Basic Beans (page 32)? Substitute 1 to 2 cups of those for the canned kidney beans.

Serving Size: 4 servings
Per Serving: Calories: 155; Total Fat: 0g; Total Carbs: 31g; Sugar: 10g; Fiber: 8g; Protein: 7g; Sodium: 1,660mg

Wild Rice Soup with Mushrooms

CORN FREE | DAIRY FREE | EGG FREE | GLUTEN FREE | NIGHTSHADE FREE | NUT FREE | SOY FREE | SUGAR FREE | VEGAN

Chicken soup with rice may be the tradition, but this entirely plant-based recipe will surprise you with its depth of flavor and absolute ease of creation. The mushrooms add a punch of unexpected protein and umami taste. Recent studies have shown that extracts from porcini mushrooms decrease markers of inflammation in the body, and therefore inhibit inflammatory disease.

SERVES 4 TO 6

Prep time: 15 minutes or fewer

Cook time: 6 to 8 hours on low

1½ cups uncooked wild rice

6 cups vegetable broth

2 carrots, diced

1 celery stalk, diced

½ medium onion, diced

¼ cup dried porcini mushrooms

1 tablespoon extra-virgin olive oil

1 teaspoon sea salt

½ teaspoon garlic powder

½ teaspoon dried thyme leaves

1 bay leaf

Freshly ground black pepper

1. In your slow cooker, combine the rice, broth, carrots, celery, onion, mushrooms, olive oil, salt, garlic powder, thyme, and bay leaf, and season with pepper.

2. Cover the cooker and set to low. Cook for 6 to 8 hours.

3. Remove and discard the bay leaf before serving.

INGREDIENT TIP: For a little bit thicker texture, stir together ¼ cup water and 2 teaspoons of arrowroot powder (a healthier alternative to cornstarch). Combine this slurry with the hot soup and stir well.

Serving Size: 4 servings
Per Serving: Calories: 425; Total Fat: 4g; Total Carbs: 78g; Sugar: 5g; Fiber: 6g; Protein: 16g; Sodium: 1,418mg

White Bean & French Onion Soup

CORN FREE | DAIRY FREE | EGG FREE | GLUTEN FREE | NIGHTSHADE FREE | NUT FREE | SOY FREE | SUGAR FREE | VEGAN

You will not miss the dripping Gruyère cheese of traditional French onion soup when you savor your first spoonful of this soup. Choose from yellow or sweet onions for this recipe, or use a bit of both. Yellow onions are bursting with flavor and end with a subtle sweetness, while sweet onions are subtler—sweet and bright toward the end. The added thyme, a miracle herb in and of itself, contains not just anti-inflammatory properties but antimicrobial, antibacterial, and potentially analgesic properties as well. In order to get perfectly caramelized onions, this recipe does require starting the onions out first, then adding in more ingredients after three hours of initial cooking time—take this into consideration as you plan your day and cooking times.

SERVES 4 TO 6

Prep time: 15 minutes or fewer

Cook time: 3 hours on high plus 4 hours on low

2 large onions, thinly sliced

¼ cup extra-virgin olive oil

¾ teaspoon sea salt

2 (14-ounce) cans cannellini beans, rinsed and drained well

4 cups vegetable broth

½ teaspoon garlic powder

½ teaspoon dried thyme leaves

1 bay leaf

Freshly ground black pepper

1. In your slow cooker, combine the onions, olive oil, and salt.

2. Cover the cooker and set to high. Cook for 3 hours, allowing the onions to caramelize.

3. Stir the onions well and add the beans, broth, garlic powder, thyme, and bay leaf, and season with pepper.

4. Re-cover the cooker and set to low. Cook for 4 hours.

5. Remove and discard the bay leaf before serving.

SERVING TIP: If you're missing the crusty bread or croutons usually served with classic soup, toast some gluten-free bread or use a traditional sourdough.

Serving Size: 4 servings
Per Serving: Calories: 328; Total Fat: 14g; Total Carbs: 39g; Sugar: 7g; Fiber: 10g; Protein: 11g; Sodium: 968mg

Spiced Sweet Potato & Almond Soup

CORN FREE | DAIRY FREE | EGG FREE | GLUTEN FREE | SOY FREE | SUGAR FREE | VEGAN

The flavor combinations in this soup are a tad unexpected but decidedly yummy! Almond butter is a great alternative to the often-inflammatory peanut butter, which can contain naturally occurring molds that can induce inflammation even if you aren't specifically allergic to peanuts.

SERVES 4 TO 6

Prep time: 15 minutes or fewer

Cook time: 6 to 8 hours on low

4 cups vegetable broth, plus more if needed (see Tip)

1 (15-ounce) can diced tomatoes

2 medium sweet potatoes, peeled and diced

1 medium onion, diced

1 jalapeño pepper, seeded and diced

½ cup unsalted almond butter

½ teaspoon sea salt

½ teaspoon garlic powder

½ teaspoon ground turmeric

½ teaspoon ground ginger

¼ teaspoon ground cinnamon

Pinch ground nutmeg

½ cup full-fat coconut milk

1. In your slow cooker, combine the broth, tomatoes, sweet potatoes, onion, jalapeño, almond butter, salt, garlic powder, turmeric, ginger, cinnamon, and nutmeg.

2. Cover the cooker and set to low. Cook for 6 to 8 hours.

3. Stir in the coconut milk after cooking.

4. Using an immersion blender, purée the soup until smooth and serve.

COOKING TIP: If you prefer a thinner soup, add a little more vegetable broth until you reach your desired consistency.

Serving Size: 4 servings
Per Serving: Calories: 358; Total Fat: 23g; Total Carbs: 34g; Sugar: 11g; Fiber: 7g; Protein: 7g; Sodium: 1,066mg

Thai Curry Vegetable Soup

CORN FREE | DAIRY FREE | EGG FREE | GLUTEN FREE | NUT FREE | SOY FREE | SUGAR FREE

Turmeric is a major player in the magical spice blend we know as curry powder. Turmeric's anti-inflammatory powers rival just about every other herb or spice on the market. It contains a component called curcumin that you can also purchase as a supplement.

SERVES 4 TO 6

Prep time: 15 minutes or fewer

Cook time: 6 to 8 hours on low

4 cups vegetable broth

½ cup sliced mushrooms

3 carrots, diced

1 bunch baby bok choy

1 sweet potato, peeled and diced

1 small head broccoli, florets chopped

1 small onion, diced

1 lemongrass stalk, chopped into 1-inch segments

1 tablespoon freshly squeezed lime juice

1 tablespoon curry paste

2 teaspoons fish sauce

¾ teaspoon sea salt

½ teaspoon ground ginger

½ teaspoon garlic powder

¾ cup full-fat coconut milk

Fresh cilantro leaves, for garnishing

1. In your slow cooker, stir together the broth, mushrooms, carrots, bok choy, sweet potato, broccoli, onion, lemongrass, lime juice, curry paste, fish sauce, salt, ginger, and garlic powder.

2. Cover the cooker and set to low. Cook for 6 to 8 hours.

3. Stir in the coconut milk and garnish with the cilantro before serving.

SUBSTITUTION TIP: In a pinch, you can substitute tamari or coconut aminos for the fish sauce. The flavor profile won't be exactly the same, but you'll still get that hit of umami flavor.

Serving Size: 4 servings
Per Serving: Calories: 229; Total Fat: 9g; Total Carbs: 31g; Sugar: 11g; Fiber: 9g; Protein: 8g; Sodium: 1,457mg

Golden Lentil Soup

CORN FREE | DAIRY FREE | EGG FREE | GLUTEN FREE | NIGHTSHADE FREE | NUT FREE | SOY FREE | SUGAR FREE | VEGAN

This soup contains the triple threat of anti-inflammatory seasonings—garlic, turmeric, and ginger. The soup gets its golden name from the turmeric, mostly, which has a potent yellow pigment that can easily stain—be careful!

SERVES 4 TO 6

Prep time: 15 minutes, plus 8 hours to soak

Cook time: 6 to 8 hours on low

1 cup dried yellow lentils, soaked in water overnight, drained, and rinsed well

4 cups vegetable broth

1 small onion, diced

1 carrot, diced

1 celery stalk, minced

2 teaspoons ground turmeric

1 teaspoon garlic powder

½ teaspoon sea salt

½ teaspoon ground ginger

½ teaspoon ground cumin

½ teaspoon dried thyme leaves

¼ teaspoon ground cinnamon

2 cups full-fat coconut milk

1. In your slow cooker, combine the lentils, broth, onion, carrot, celery, turmeric, garlic, salt, ginger, cumin, thyme, and cinnamon.

2. Cover the cooker and set to low. Cook for 6 to 8 hours.

3. Stir in the coconut milk and serve.

INGREDIENT TIP: Add a little green to this golden soup. Roughly chop 1 cup of fresh spinach and stir it in after the cooking time is done, allowing it to wilt into the warmth of the soup. When you add spinach to a warm dish, the extra cooking means your body can better absorb the spinach's antioxidants, such as vitamins A and E, zinc, thiamin, and calcium.

Serving Size: 4 servings
Per Serving: Calories: 328; Total Fat: 21g; Total Carbs: 32g; Sugar: 7g; Fiber: 13g; Protein: 12g; Sodium: 876mg

Zuppa Toscana

CORN FREE | DAIRY FREE | EGG FREE | GLUTEN FREE | NUT FREE | SOY FREE | SUGAR FREE | VEGAN

Zucchini contains high percentages of beta-carotene, vitamin C, and copper, which are all known to have anti-inflammatory properties that can help reduce symptoms of inflammatory diseases, such as arthritis. To keep this classic soup plant based, I've omitted the Italian bacon, but you won't miss it after tasting the powerhouse of other flavors in this dish.

SERVES 4 TO 6

Prep time: 15 minutes or fewer

Cook time: 5 to 6 hours on low

4 cups vegetable broth

2 cups chopped de-ribbed kale

2 small sweet potatoes, peeled and diced

1 medium zucchini, diced

1 (15-ounce) can cannellini beans, rinsed and drained well

1 celery stalk, diced

1 carrot, diced

1 small onion, diced

½ teaspoon garlic powder

½ teaspoon sea salt

¼ teaspoon red pepper flakes

Freshly ground black pepper

1. In your slow cooker, combine the broth, kale, sweet potatoes, zucchini, beans, celery, carrot, onion, garlic powder, salt, and red pepper flakes, and season with black pepper.

2. Cover the cooker and set to low. Cook for 5 to 6 hours and serve.

TIME-SAVING TIP: Use a bag of frozen cubed sweet potatoes for this recipe. Just be sure to thaw in the refrigerator the night before adding them to the slow cooker, or the timing and temperature of the dish will be off.

Serving Size: 4 servings
Per Serving: Calories: 209; Total Fat: 1g; Total Carbs: 43g; Sugar: 9g; Fiber: 10g; Protein: 8g; Sodium: 871mg

Turmeric-Broccoli Soup

CORN FREE | DAIRY FREE | EGG FREE | GLUTEN FREE | NIGHTSHADE FREE | NUT FREE | SOY FREE | SUGAR FREE | VEGAN

Out of all foods, broccoli has the fifth highest levels of folate, which is extremely important for healthy cell growth and function. This soup displays the broccoli well, boasting of many herbs and spices to both lower inflammation and make it taste amazing.

SERVES 4 TO 6

Prep time: 15 minutes or fewer

Cook time: 3 to 4 hours on low

2 medium heads broccoli

½ medium onion, diced

1 tablespoon extra-virgin olive oil

1 tablespoon ground turmeric

½ teaspoon garlic powder

½ teaspoon ground ginger

1 teaspoon freshly squeezed lemon juice

½ teaspoon sea salt

4 cups vegetable broth

Freshly ground black pepper

1. In your slow cooker, combine the broccoli, onion, olive oil, turmeric, garlic powder, ginger, lemon juice, salt, and broth, and season with pepper.

2. Cover the cooker and set to low. Cook for 3 to 4 hours and serve.

SERVING TIP: You can purée the slow cooker contents with an immersion blender for a much thicker base.

Serving Size: 4 servings
Per Serving: Calories: 144; Total Fat: 5g; Total Carbs: 22g; Sugar: 8g; Fiber: 11g; Protein: 9g; Sodium: 904mg

Indian-Spiced Cauliflower

CORN FREE | DAIRY FREE | EGG FREE | GLUTEN FREE | NUT FREE | SOY FREE | SUGAR FREE | VEGAN

Cauliflower is extremely high in the antioxidant vitamin C. Interestingly, recent studies have shown that cooked versus raw cauliflower has many benefits, including the ability to bind to bile salts and help with detoxification in that way. It is also linked to better regulation of blood cholesterol.

SERVES 4 TO 6

Prep time: 15 minutes or fewer

Cook time: 3 to 4 hours on low

1 large head cauliflower, leaves and large stem removed

½ medium onion, diced

2 tablespoons extra-virgin olive oil

½ teaspoon sea salt

½ teaspoon garlic powder

½ teaspoon ground ginger

½ teaspoon curry powder

¼ teaspoon ground turmeric

¼ teaspoon ground cumin

⅛ teaspoon cayenne pepper

1. Chop the cauliflower into florets, and place them in the slow cooker with the onion.

2. In a small bowl, combine the olive oil, salt, garlic powder, ginger, curry powder, turmeric, cumin, and cayenne. Whisk into a paste. Using a pastry brush or a spoon, spread the spice paste onto the cauliflower florets.

3. Cover the cooker and set to low. Cook for 3 to 4 hours and serve.

TIME-SAVING TIP: Look for bagged cauliflower florets at the grocery store to save time prepping and chopping.

Serving Size: 4 servings
Per Serving: Calories: 121; Total Fat: 7g; Total Carbs: 13g; Sugar: 5g; Fiber: 6g; Protein: 4g; Sodium: 354mg

Maple-Dijon Brussels Sprouts

CORN FREE | DAIRY FREE | EGG FREE | GLUTEN FREE | NIGHTSHADE FREE | NUT FREE | SOY FREE | VEGAN

Brussels sprouts are extremely high in antioxidants and contain compounds that may help lower inflammation levels. These little green sprouts used to be the butt of many "gross food" jokes, but now they're seen on almost every trendy restaurant menu as the most popular appetizer or side. Make your own at home for lunch or a side at dinner.

SERVES 4 TO 6

Prep time: 15 minutes or fewer

Cook time: 3 to 4 hours on low

1 pound Brussels sprouts, ends trimmed

2 tablespoons maple syrup

1 tablespoon Dijon mustard

½ teaspoon garlic powder

½ teaspoon sea salt

¼ cup water

1. In your slow cooker, combine the Brussels sprouts, maple syrup, mustard, garlic powder, salt, and water. Toss together to distribute evenly.

2. Cover the cooker and set to low. Cook for 3 to 4 hours and serve.

INGREDIENT TIP: Grate a little raw sheep's milk pecorino cheese (similar to Parmesan) on top of the sprouts while they're still warm for an extra treat if your body tolerates dairy.

Serving Size: 4 servings
Per Serving: Calories: 80; Total Fat: 0g; Total Carbs: 17g; Sugar: 9g; Fiber: 4g; Protein: 4g; Sodium: 410mg

Balsamic Beets

CORN FREE | DAIRY FREE | EGG FREE | GLUTEN FREE | NIGHTSHADE FREE | NUT FREE | SOY FREE | VEGAN

Beets are arguably the perfect food for the anti-inflammatory diet. This root veggie with incredible cleansing power includes compounds called betains, which help the cells in the liver eliminate toxins, as well as pigments called betalains, which rank extremely high for their overall anti-inflammatory properties.

SERVES 4 TO 6

Prep time: 15 minutes or fewer

Cook time: 6 to 8 hours on low

4 to 6 medium beets (they need to fit snugly in the bottom of your slow cooker), chopped (see Tip)

½ cup balsamic vinegar

1 cup apple juice

½ teaspoon garlic powder

½ teaspoon dried rosemary

Freshly ground black pepper

1. In your slow cooker, combine the beets, vinegar, apple juice, garlic powder, and rosemary, and season with pepper.

2. Cover the cooker and set to low. Cook for 6 to 8 hours and serve.

PREPARATION TIP: I prefer to peel my beets, but you don't have to. Just remember to wash and scrub them well if you're going to leave them unpeeled.

Serving Size: 4 servings
Per Serving: Calories: 96; Total Fat: 0g; Total Carbs: 21g; Sugar: 13g; Fiber: 1g; Protein: 0g; Sodium: 87mg

Kale & White Bean Chili

CORN FREE | DAIRY FREE | EGG FREE | GLUTEN FREE | NUT FREE | SOY FREE | SUGAR FREE | VEGAN

This is one hearty and protein-packed chili. Add more broth and cut out the chili powder in this recipe to make a smooth and healthy bean soup if you're not a chili fan. Either way, this recipe provides perfect leftovers for lunch the following day, or even the day after!

SERVES 4 TO 6

Prep time: 15 minutes, plus 8 hours to soak

Cook time: 6 to 8 hours on low

2 cups dried cannellini beans, soaked in water overnight, drained, and rinsed well

1 small bunch kale, washed, chopped, and de-ribbed

1 small onion, diced

½ green bell pepper, seeded and chopped

1 (4-ounce) can Hatch green chiles

4 cups vegetable broth

½ teaspoon garlic powder

1 teaspoon chili powder

½ teaspoon ground cumin

2 tablespoons extra-virgin olive oil

1 avocado, peeled, pitted, and chopped

1. In your slow cooker, combine the beans, kale, onion, bell pepper, chiles, broth, garlic powder, chili powder, and cumin. Stir to mix the ingredients.

2. Cover the cooker and set to low. Cook for 6 to 8 hours.

3. Drizzle each bowl with olive oil, top with avocado, and serve.

TIME-SAVING TIP: Look for precut kale in bags at your grocery store to save time chopping, washing, and removing the stems and ribs.

Serving Size: 4 servings

Per Serving: Calories: 476; Total Fat: 16g; Total Carbs: 67g; Sugar: 3g; Fiber: 13g; Protein: 22g; Sodium: 589mg

Lentil Bolognese

CORN FREE | DAIRY FREE | EGG FREE | GLUTEN FREE | NUT FREE | SOY FREE | SUGAR FREE | VEGAN

Serve this chunky, delicious, and protein-rich sauce over a bed of brown rice pasta, or eat it by itself! Lentils provide a wealth of fiber to keep your digestive tract cleansed and operating well. To get the best flavor out of the carrots, celery, and onion, this recipe does require starting those ingredients out first, then adding in more ingredients after 30 minutes of initial cooking time—take this into consideration as you plan your day and cooking times.

SERVES 4 TO 6

Prep time: 15 minutes, plus 8 hours to soak

Cook time: 30 minutes on high plus 5 to 6 hours on low

1 tablespoon extra-virgin olive oil

2 carrots, grated

1 celery stalk, minced

1 small onion, diced

½ teaspoon garlic powder

4 cups diced tomatoes

2 cups vegetable broth

1 cup lentils, soaked in water overnight, drained, and rinsed well

1 bay leaf

½ teaspoon dried oregano

½ teaspoon dried basil leaves

½ teaspoon sea salt

¼ teaspoon red pepper flakes

¼ teaspoon ground nutmeg

Freshly ground black pepper

1. Coat the slow cooker with the olive oil. Add the carrots, celery, onion, and garlic powder.

2. Cover the cooker and set to high. Cook for 30 minutes.

3. Stir in the tomatoes, broth, lentils, bay leaf, oregano, basil, salt, red pepper flakes, and nutmeg, then season with black pepper. Re-cover the cooker and set to low. Cook for 5 to 6 hours.

4. Remove and discard the bay leaf before serving.

INGREDIENT TIP: As with many of these recipes, you can add some secret greens by mincing 1 cup of fresh spinach and stirring it into the lentils to wilt at the end of the cooking time.

Serving Size: 4 servings
Per Serving: Calories: 180; Total Fat: 4g; Total Carbs: 35g; Sugar: 5g; Fiber: 15g; Protein: 12g; Sodium: 607mg

Masala Lentils

CORN FREE | DAIRY FREE | EGG FREE | GLUTEN FREE | NUT FREE | SOY FREE | VEGAN

When it comes to spices, masala is essentially any of the many spice mixes used in South Asian cuisine. Garam masala, on the other hand, hails specifically from India and typically contains black pepper, clove, cinnamon, nutmeg, coriander, bay, cumin, and cardamom. Many of these spices are used in Ayurvedic medicine to heat the body and heal it.

SERVES 4 TO 6

Prep time: 15 minutes, plus 8 hours to soak

Cook time: 4 to 5 hours on low

1 cup red lentils, soaked in water overnight, drained, and rinsed well

1 (15-ounce) can diced tomatoes

1 medium onion, diced

2 cups vegetable broth

2 teaspoons garam masala

1 teaspoon garlic powder

1 teaspoon ground ginger

1 teaspoon molasses

1 teaspoon sea salt

½ teaspoon paprika

½ teaspoon ground turmeric

Pinch cayenne pepper

Freshly ground black pepper

1 cup fresh spinach, roughly chopped

1 cup full-fat coconut milk

1. In your slow cooker, combine the lentils, tomatoes, onion, broth, garam masala, garlic powder, ginger, molasses, salt, paprika, turmeric, and cayenne, and season with black pepper.

2. Cover the cooker and set to low. Cook for 4 to 5 hours.

3. Stir in the spinach and re-cover the cooker for 5 minutes to let the spinach wilt.

4. Add the coconut milk, stir, and serve.

INGREDIENT TIP: Because of its complexity, if you don't have garam masala in your pantry, it's hard to replicate perfectly. Thankfully, though, you could easily substitute one part cumin and one-fourth part allspice.

Serving Size: 4 servings

Per Serving: Calories: 232; Total Fat: 11g; Total Carbs: 32g; Sugar: 8g; Fiber: 13g; Protein: 12g; Sodium: 1,095mg

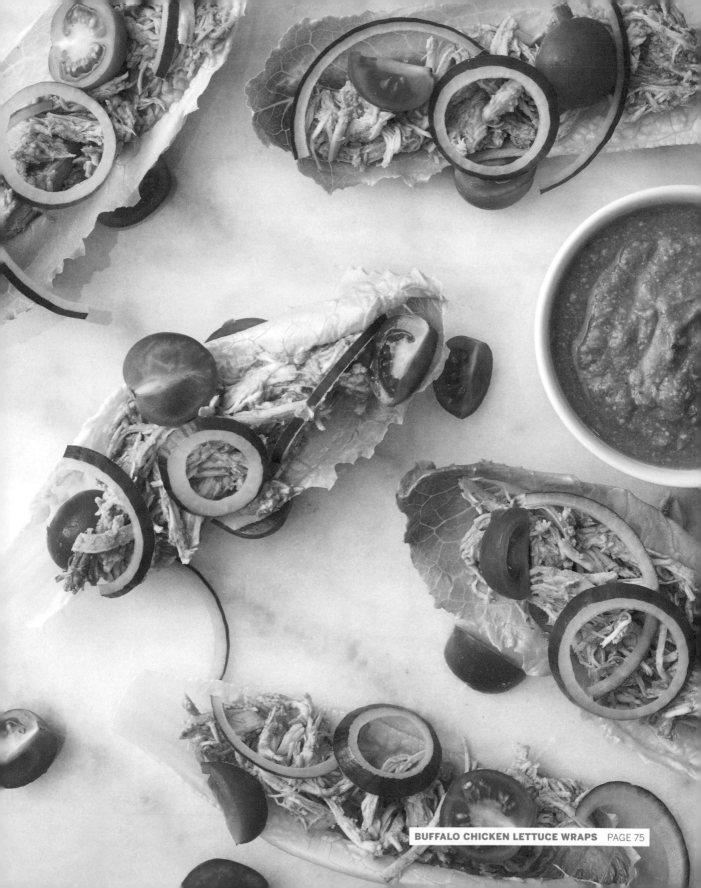

BUFFALO CHICKEN LETTUCE WRAPS PAGE 75

5 | POULTRY

Chicken Bone Broth

CORN FREE | DAIRY FREE | EGG FREE | GLUTEN FREE | NIGHTSHADE FREE | NUT FREE | SOY FREE | SUGAR FREE

Bone broths, in general, are very high in the anti-inflammatory amino acids glycine and proline. Glucosamine is a compound found in connective tissue, which has been shown to reduce pain and inflammation. And chicken bones are so packed with nutrients that you can actually turn this recipe into a "perpetual recipe" if you have the time. Rather than stopping the process after 6 to 8 hours, simply ladle the liquid from the slow cooker through a sieve and into jars, leaving the ingredients in the slow cooker and adding more water to cover them for another round of cooking.

MAKES ABOUT 12 CUPS

Prep time: 15 minutes or fewer

Cook time: 6 to 8 hours on low

1 chicken carcass

About 12 cups filtered water (enough to cover the bones)

2 carrots, roughly chopped

2 garlic cloves, roughly chopped

1 celery stalk, roughly chopped

½ onion, roughly chopped

2 bay leaves

1 parsley sprig

¾ teaspoon sea salt

½ teaspoon dried oregano

½ teaspoon dried basil leaves

1 tablespoon apple cider vinegar

1. In your slow cooker, combine the chicken carcass, water, carrots, garlic, celery, onion, bay leaves, parsley, salt, oregano, basil, and vinegar.

2. Cover the cooker and set to low. Cook for 6 to 8 hours.

3. Skim off any scum from the surface of the broth, and pour the broth through a fine-mesh sieve into a large bowl, discarding the chicken and veggie scraps. Refrigerate the broth in an airtight container for up to 5 days, or freeze it for up to 3 months.

INGREDIENT TIP: The apple cider vinegar may sound out of place, but it actually helps leach more nutrients from the chicken bones and into your broth. Don't skip it!

Serving Size: 1 cup
Per Serving: Calories: 50; Total Fat: 1g; Total Carbs: 1g; Sugar: 0g; Fiber: 0g; Protein: 9g; Sodium: 145mg

Basic "Rotisserie" Chicken

CORN FREE | DAIRY FREE | EGG FREE | GLUTEN FREE | NUT FREE | SOY FREE | SUGAR FREE

Making a whole cooked chicken at the beginning of the week is one of the best ways you can simplify meal prep. You can use the different chicken pieces for different meals on different days. And don't forget to save your chicken carcass and bones for making Chicken Bone Broth (page 68)!

SERVES 4 TO 6

Prep time: 15 minutes or fewer

Cook time: 6 to 8 hours on low

1 teaspoon garlic powder

1 teaspoon chili powder

1 teaspoon paprika

1 teaspoon dried thyme leaves

1 teaspoon sea salt

Pinch cayenne pepper

Freshly ground black pepper

1 whole chicken (about 4 to 5 pounds), neck and giblets removed

½ medium onion, sliced

1. In a small bowl, stir together the garlic powder, chili powder, paprika, thyme, salt, and cayenne. Season with black pepper, and stir again to combine. Rub the spice mix all over the exterior of the chicken.

2. Place the chicken in the slow cooker with the sliced onion sprinkled around it.

3. Cover the cooker and set to low. Cook for 6 to 8 hours, or until the internal temperature reaches 165°F on a meat thermometer and the juices run clear, and serve.

SERVING TIP: You can crisp the skin to mimic a true rotisserie chicken by popping your finished chicken under your oven's preheated broiler for 3 to 5 minutes.

Serving Size: 4 servings
Per Serving: Calories: 862; Total Fat: 59g; Total Carbs: 7g; Sugar:6 g; Fiber: 0g; Protein: 86g; Sodium: 1,200mg

Tangy Barbecue Chicken

CORN FREE | DAIRY FREE | EGG FREE | NUT FREE

Studies have shown there is a positive change in the composition of a person's blood level triglycerides with chicken consumption due to the anti-inflammatory omega-3 fatty acids it provides. This shredded barbecue chicken dish can be served myriad ways: plain, over rice, on a gluten-free bun, over a salad—the list goes on! You can make the barbecue sauce ahead of time or throw the sauce ingredients together at the time you're cooking the chicken.

SERVES 4 TO 6

Prep time: 15 minutes or fewer

Cook time: 3 to 4 hours on high

4 to 5 boneless, skinless chicken breasts (about 2 pounds; see Tip)

2 cups Tangy Barbecue Sauce with Apple Cider Vinegar (page 113)

1. In your slow cooker, combine the chicken and barbecue sauce. Stir until the chicken breasts are well coated in the sauce.

2. Cover the cooker and set to high. Cook for 3 to 4 hours, or until the internal temperature of the chicken reaches 165°F on a meat thermometer and the juices run clear.

3. Shred the chicken with a fork, mix it into the sauce, and serve.

SAFETY TIP: Don't rinse or wash your chicken beforehand! This is an old, but popular, myth. In truth, rinsing raw chicken only serves to spread potentially harmful bacteria throughout your kitchen.

Serving Size: 4 servings
Per Serving: Calories: 412; Total Fat: 13g; Total Carbs: 22g; Sugar: 19g; Fiber: 0g; Protein: 51g; Sodium: 766mg

Salsa Verde Chicken

CORN FREE | DAIRY FREE | EGG FREE | GLUTEN FREE | NUT FREE | SOY FREE | SUGAR FREE

Reignite taco night with this fork-tender pulled chicken. You're in control of the spice, depending on which favorite green salsa you choose. The proof that flavor doesn't need to be inflammatory is found in this dish!

SERVES 4 TO 6

Prep time: 15 minutes or fewer

Cook time: 6 to 8 hours on low

4 to 5 boneless, skinless chicken breasts (about 2 pounds)

2 cups green salsa

1 cup chicken broth

2 tablespoons freshly squeezed lime juice

1 teaspoon sea salt

1 teaspoon chili powder

1. In your slow cooker, combine the chicken, salsa, broth, lime juice, salt, and chili powder. Stir to combine.

2. Cover the cooker and set to low. Cook for 6 to 8 hours, or until the internal temperature of the chicken reaches 165°F on a meat thermometer and the juices run clear.

3. Shred the chicken with a fork, mix it into the sauce, and serve.

INGREDIENT TIP: When choosing a green salsa, you'll find they typically have tomatillos listed as the main ingredient. This is excellent, considering that tomatillos have the ability to fight inflammation and prevent cancer growth.

Serving Size: 4 servings
Per Serving: Calories: 318; Total Fat: 8g; Total Carbs: 6g; Sugar: 2g; Fiber: 1g; Protein: 52g; Sodium: 1,510mg

Lemon & Garlic Chicken Thighs

CORN FREE | DAIRY FREE | EGG FREE | GLUTEN FREE | NIGHTSHADE FREE | NUT FREE | SOY FREE | SUGAR FREE

Even though it's very acidic, consuming lemon juice on a daily basis can help alkalize the acidity in your body, thereby decreasing inflammation. I love adding it to water, desserts, soups, and even chicken!

SERVES 4 TO 6

Prep time: 15 minutes or fewer

Cook time: 7 to 8 hours on low

2 cups chicken broth

1½ teaspoons garlic powder

1 teaspoon sea salt

Juice and zest of
1 large lemon

2 pounds boneless skinless
chicken thighs

1. Pour the broth into the slow cooker.

2. In a small bowl, stir together the garlic powder, salt, lemon juice, and lemon zest. Baste each chicken thigh with an even coating of the mixture. Place the thighs along the bottom of the slow cooker.

3. Cover the cooker and set to low. Cook for 7 to 8 hours, or until the internal temperature of the chicken reaches 165°F on a meat thermometer and the juices run clear, and serve.

COOKING TIP: If you have time, adding 4 or 5 minced garlic cloves punches up the flavor and contributes powerful anti-inflammatory benefits.

TECHNIQUE TIP: If only skin-on thighs are available, you can still use them to make this recipe. For a more appetizing finish and to seal in the juices, add a quick stove top step by searing the thighs first. Heat a skillet on medium-high. Add 1 tablespoon of avocado oil and place the chicken skin-side down. Sear for 10 minutes, or until the skin is brown, and remove from the heat. Proceed to Step 1 of the recipe.

Serving Size: 4 servings
Per Serving: Calories: 290; Total Fat: 14g; Total Carbs: 3g; Sugar: 0g; Fiber: 0g; Protein: 43g; Sodium: 1,017mg

Slow Cooker Chicken Fajitas

CORN FREE | DAIRY FREE | EGG FREE | GLUTEN FREE | NUT FREE | SOY FREE | SUGAR FREE

Capsaicin is the compound in peppers that makes them hot. It's also thought to decrease inflammation in the body, as it has been shown to relieve pain by causing the body to release endorphins. In this recipe you'll find a wealth of different peppers, all providing innumerable health benefits, heat, and flavor.

SERVES 4 TO 6

Prep time: 15 minutes or fewer

Cook time: 7 to 8 hours on low

1 (14.5-ounce) can diced tomatoes

1 (4-ounce) can Hatch green chiles

1½ teaspoons garlic powder

2 teaspoons chili powder

1½ teaspoons ground cumin

1 teaspoon paprika

1 teaspoon sea salt

Juice of 1 lime

Pinch cayenne pepper

Freshly ground black pepper

1 red bell pepper, seeded and sliced

1 green bell pepper, seeded and sliced

1 yellow bell pepper, seeded and sliced

1 large onion, sliced

2 pounds boneless, skinless chicken breast

1. In a medium bowl, combine the diced tomatoes, chiles, garlic powder, chili powder, cumin, paprika, salt, lime juice, and cayenne, and season with black pepper. Mix well. Pour half the diced tomato mixture into the bottom of your slow cooker.

2. Layer half the red, green, and yellow bell peppers and half the onion over the tomatoes in the cooker.

3. Place the chicken on top of the peppers and onions.

4. Cover the chicken with the remaining red, green, and yellow bell peppers and onions. Pour the remaining tomato mixture on top.

5. Cover the cooker and set to low. Cook for 7 to 8 hours, or until the internal temperature of the chicken reaches 165°F on a meat thermometer and the juices run clear, and serve.

SERVING TIP: While fajitas are traditionally served with flour or corn tortillas, you can easily serve this dish over a bowl of hearty grains, such as brown rice or quinoa.

Serving Size: 4 servings
Per Serving: Calories: 310; Total Fat: 5g; Total Carbs: 19g; Sugar: 7g; Fiber: 4g; Protein: 46g; Sodium: 1,541mg

White Bean, Chicken & Apple Cider Chili

CORN FREE | DAIRY FREE | EGG FREE | GLUTEN FREE | NUT FREE | SOY FREE | SUGAR FREE

Apple cider vinegar's alkaline pH helps bring the body to a place of health and healing while adding a zingy and unexpected kick to this autumnal chili recipe.

SERVES 4 TO 6

Prep time: 15 minutes or fewer

Cook time: 7 to 8 hours on low

3 cups chopped cooked chicken (see Basic "Rotisserie" Chicken, page 69)

2 (15-ounce) cans white navy beans, rinsed well and drained

1 medium onion, chopped

1 (15-ounce) can diced tomatoes

3 cups Chicken Bone Broth (page 68) or store-bought chicken broth

1 cup apple cider

2 bay leaves

1 tablespoon extra-virgin olive oil

2 teaspoons garlic powder

1 teaspoon chili powder

1 teaspoon sea salt

½ teaspoon ground cumin

¼ teaspoon ground cinnamon

Pinch cayenne pepper

Freshly ground black pepper

¼ cup apple cider vinegar

1. In your slow cooker, combine the chicken, beans, onion, tomatoes, broth, cider, bay leaves, olive oil, garlic powder, chili powder, salt, cumin, cinnamon, and cayenne, and season with black pepper.

2. Cover the cooker and set to low. Cook for 7 to 8 hours.

3. Remove and discard the bay leaves. Stir in the apple cider vinegar until well blended and serve.

INGREDIENT TIP: Because we're adding the vinegar at the end, we aren't overcooking its life-giving enzymes and probiotics. Choose a raw, unfiltered apple cider vinegar to reap all the benefits of this ancient tonic.

Serving Size: 4 servings
Per Serving: Calories: 469; Total Fat: 8g; Total Carbs: 46g; Sugar: 13g; Fiber: 9g; Protein: 51g; Sodium: 1,047mg

Buffalo Chicken Lettuce Wraps

CORN FREE | DAIRY FREE | EGG FREE | GLUTEN FREE | SOY FREE | SUGAR FREE

Choosing to use leafy greens instead of wheat products is always an anti-inflammatory win! Your body will thank you for the light, refreshing replacement of a roll with the romaine lettuce leaves here.

SERVES 4 TO 6

Prep time: 15 minutes or fewer

Cook time: 7 to 8 hours on low

1 tablespoon extra-virgin olive oil

2 pounds boneless, skinless chicken breast

2 cups Vegan Buffalo Dip (page 116)

1 cup water

8 to 10 romaine lettuce leaves

½ red onion, thinly sliced

1 cup cherry tomatoes, halved

1. Coat the bottom of the slow cooker with the olive oil.

2. Add the chicken, dip, and water, and stir to combine.

3. Cover the cooker and set to low. Cook for 7 to 8 hours, or until the internal temperature of the chicken reaches 165°F on a meat thermometer and the juices run clear.

4. Shred the chicken with a fork, and mix it into the dip in the slow cooker.

5. Divide the meat mixture among the lettuce leaves. Top with onion and tomato, and serve.

INGREDIENT TIP: Try other sturdy green vegetable leaves instead of romaine for different nutrient profiles. Good options to start with include chard or collard greens.

Serving Sizze: 4 servings

Per Serving: Calories. 437; Total Fat: 18g; Total Carbs: 18g; Sugar: 8g; Fiber: 4g; Protein: 49g; Sodium: 993mg

Cilantro-Lime Chicken Drumsticks

CORN FREE | DAIRY FREE | EGG FREE | GLUTEN FREE | NIGHTSHADE FREE | NUT FREE | SOY FREE | SUGAR FREE

Coriander seed, which grows into the cilantro plant, is well established as an anti-inflammatory herb and commonly believed to aid digestion as well. Save a few fresh leaves to sprinkle on top before serving.

SERVES 4 TO 6

Prep time: 15 minutes or fewer

Cook time: 2 to 3 hours on high

¼ cup fresh cilantro, chopped

3 tablespoons freshly squeezed lime juice

½ teaspoon garlic powder

½ teaspoon sea salt

¼ teaspoon ground cumin

3 pounds chicken drumsticks

1. In a small bowl, stir together the cilantro, lime juice, garlic powder, salt, and cumin to form a paste.

2. Put the drumsticks in the slow cooker. Spread the cilantro paste evenly on each drumstick.

3. Cover the cooker and set to high. Cook for 2 to 3 hours, or until the internal temperature of the chicken reaches 165°F on a meat thermometer and the juices run clear, and serve (see Tip).

COOKING TIP: To crisp the drumsticks before serving, place them under your oven's preheated broiler for 5 minutes.

Serving Size: 4 servings
Per Serving: Calories: 417; Total Fat: 12g; Total Carbs: 1g; Sugar: 1g; Fiber: 1g; Protein: 71g; Sodium: 591mg

Coconut-Curry-Cashew Chicken

Curry powder contains some powerful antioxidants and anti-inflammatory compounds. The oils in lemongrass, a main ingredient in red curry paste, are known to have antifungal, insecticidal, antiseptic, and anti-inflammatory properties.

SERVES 4 TO 6

Prep time: 15 minutes or fewer

Cook time: 7 to 8 hours on low

1½ cups Chicken Bone Broth (page 68)

1 (14-ounce) can full-fat coconut milk

1 teaspoon garlic powder

1 tablespoon red curry paste

1 teaspoon sea salt

½ teaspoon freshly ground black pepper

½ teaspoon coconut sugar

2 pounds boneless, skinless chicken breasts

1½ cup unsalted cashews

½ cup diced white onion

1. In a medium bowl, combine the broth, coconut milk, garlic powder, red curry paste, salt, pepper, and coconut sugar. Stir well.

2. Put the chicken, cashews, and onion in the slow cooker. Pour the coconut milk, mixture on top.

3. Cover the cooker and set to low. Cook for 7 to 8 hours, or until the internal temperature of the chicken reaches 165°F on a meat thermometer and the juices run clear.

4. Shred the chicken with a fork, and mix it into the cooking liquid. You can also remove the chicken from the broth and chop it with a knife into bite-size pieces before returning it to the slow cooker. Serve.

INGREDIENT TIP: If you're looking for more flavor and a thicker broth, add 1 to 2 tablespoons of tomato paste with the curry paste.

Serving Size: 4 servings
Per Serving: Calories: 714; Total Fat: 43g; Total Carbs: 21g; Sugar: 5g; Fiber: 3g; Protein: 57g; Sodium: 1,606mg

Turkey & Sweet Potato Chili

CORN FREE | DAIRY FREE | EGG FREE | GLUTEN FREE | NUT FREE | SOY FREE | SUGAR FREE

The red onion in this chili not only adds a burst of flavor but is naturally high in the potent antioxidant quercetin, which helps the body fight inflammation. This warm, beanless chili is the perfect anti-inflammatory weeknight dinner. For toppings, try some slices of avocado, sliced scallions, and fresh cilantro leaves.

SERVES 4 TO 6

Prep time: 15 minutes or fewer

Cook time: 4 to 6 hours on low

1 tablespoon extra-virgin olive oil

1 pound ground turkey

3 cups sweet potato cubes

1 (28-ounce) can diced tomatoes

1 red bell pepper, diced

1 (4-ounce) can Hatch green chiles

½ medium red onion, diced

2 cups broth of choice

1 tablespoon freshly squeezed lime juice

1 tablespoon chili powder

1 teaspoon garlic powder

1 teaspoon cocoa powder

1 teaspoon ground cumin

1 teaspoon sea salt

½ teaspoon ground cinnamon

Pinch cayenne pepper

1. In your slow cooker, combine the olive oil, turkey, sweet potato cubes, tomatoes, bell pepper, chiles, onion, broth, lime juice, chili powder, garlic powder, cocoa powder, cumin, salt, cinnamon, and cayenne. Using a large spoon, break up the turkey into smaller chunks as it combines with the other ingredients.

2. Cover the cooker and set to low. Cook for 4 to 6 hours.

3. Stir the chili well, continuing to break up the rest of the turkey, and serve.

TIME-SAVING TIP: Grab a bag of frozen precut sweet potato chunks and thaw them in the refrigerator the night before so you don't have to peel and chop fresh ones.

Serving Size: 4 servings
Per Serving: Calories: 380; Total Fat: 12g; Total Carbs: 38g; Sugar: 12g; Fiber: 6g; Protein: 30g; Sodium: 1,268mg

Moroccan Turkey Tagine

CORN FREE | DAIRY FREE | EGG FREE | GLUTEN FREE | NUT FREE | SOY FREE

Tagine recipes typically include a spice blend called *ras el hanout*, which is uncommon in most American kitchens. While there is no one recipe for this North African spice blend, I've included many of its constituents in this tagine, and I love how they all work to lower inflammation in the body.

SERVES 4 TO 6

Prep time: 15 minutes or fewer

Cook time: 7 to 8 hours on low

4 cups boneless, skinless turkey breast chunks

1 (14-ounce) can diced tomatoes

1 (14-ounce) can chickpeas, rinsed and drained well

2 large carrots, finely chopped

½ cup dried apricots

½ red onion, chopped

2 tablespoons raw honey

1 tablespoon tomato paste

1 teaspoon garlic powder

1 teaspoon ground turmeric

½ teaspoon sea salt

¼ teaspoon ground ginger

¼ teaspoon ground coriander

¼ teaspoon paprika

½ cup water

2 cups broth of choice

Freshly ground black pepper

1. In your slow cooker, combine the turkey, tomatoes, chickpeas, carrots, apricots, onion, honey, tomato paste, garlic powder, turmeric, salt, ginger, coriander, paprika, water, and broth, and season with pepper. Gently stir to blend the ingredients.

2. Cover the cooker and set to low. Cook for 7 to 8 hours and serve.

SERVING TIP: To add even more veggies into your dinner, serve this tagine over a bed of warmed cauliflower rice.

Serving Size: 4 servings

Per Serving: Calories: 428; Total Fat: 5g; Total Carbs: 46g; Sugar: 25g; Fiber: 8g; Protein: 49g; Sodium: 983mg

Turkey Sloppy Joes

CORN FREE | DAIRY FREE | EGG FREE | GLUTEN FREE | NUT FREE | SOY FREE

Apple cider vinegar has an alkaline pH, which aids in balancing out our bodies' acidity levels and reducing inflammation quickly. Make this twist on a childhood classic unique to you by adding jalapeño peppers, different natural sweeteners (such as raw honey), and an array of spices.

SERVES 4 TO 6

Prep time: 15 minutes or fewer

Cook time: 4 to 6 hours on low

1 tablespoon extra-virgin olive oil

1 pound ground turkey

1 celery stalk, minced

1 carrot, minced

½ medium sweet onion, diced

½ red bell pepper, finely chopped

6 tablespoons tomato paste

2 tablespoons apple cider vinegar

1 tablespoon maple syrup

1 teaspoon Dijon mustard

1 teaspoon chili powder

½ teaspoon garlic powder

½ teaspoon sea salt

½ teaspoon dried oregano

1. In your slow cooker, combine the olive oil, turkey, celery, carrot, onion, red bell pepper, tomato paste, vinegar, maple syrup, mustard, chili powder, garlic powder, salt, and oregano. Using a large spoon, break up the turkey into smaller chunks as it combines with the other ingredients.

2. Cover the cooker and set to low. Cook for 4 to 6 hours, stir thoroughly, and serve.

SERVING TIP: Serve this tasty sloppy joe mixture alone, over a leafy green salad, or with gluten-free bread or rice cakes.

Serving Size: 4 servings
Per Serving: Calories: 251; Total Fat: 12g; Total Carbs: 14g; Sugar: 9g; Fiber: 3g; Protein: 24g; Sodium: 690mg

Turkey Meatballs with Spaghetti Squash

CORN FREE | DAIRY FREE | GLUTEN FREE | NUT FREE | SOY FREE | SUGAR FREE

I love this recipe because it's essentially three separate pieces of a meal, all cooked in one pot … your slow cooker! You don't have to bake the meatballs separately or dirty more pans on the stove for the spaghetti squash. If you have it on hand, adding fresh basil to the sauce after cooking will add more anti-inflammatory power plus an undeniable flavor lift.

SERVES 4 TO 6

Prep time: 15 minutes or fewer

Cook time: 6 to 7 hours on low

1 spaghetti squash, halved lengthwise and seeded

FOR THE SAUCE

1 (15-ounce) can diced tomatoes

½ teaspoon garlic powder

½ teaspoon dried oregano

½ teaspoon sea salt

FOR THE MEATBALLS

1 pound ground turkey

1 large egg, whisked

½ small white onion, minced

1 teaspoon garlic powder

½ teaspoon sea salt

½ teaspoon dried oregano

½ teaspoon dried basil leaves

Freshly ground black pepper

TO BEGIN

Place the squash halves in the bottom of your slow cooker, cut-side down.

TO MAKE THE SAUCE

1. Pour the diced tomatoes around the squash in the bottom of the slow cooker.

2. Sprinkle in the garlic powder, oregano, and salt.

TO MAKE THE MEATBALLS

1. In a medium bowl, mix together the turkey, egg, onion, garlic powder, salt, oregano, and basil, and season with pepper. Form the turkey mixture into 12 balls, and place them in the slow cooker around the spaghetti squash.

2. Cover the cooker and set to low. Cook for 6 to 7 hours.

3. Transfer the squash to a work surface, and use a fork to shred it into spaghetti-like strands. Combine the strands with the tomato sauce, top with the meatballs, and serve.

INGREDIENT TIP: For added texture and flavor, add 1 slice gluten-free bread (torn into pieces) to the turkey meatball mixture before forming it into meatballs.

Serving Size: 4 servings

Per Serving: Calories: 253; Total Fat: 8g; Total Carbs: 22g; Sugar: 4g; Fiber: 1g; Protein: 24g; Sodium: 948mg

Chimichurri Turkey & Green Beans

CORN FREE | DAIRY FREE | EGG FREE | GLUTEN FREE | NIGHTSHADE FREE | NUT FREE | SOY FREE | SUGAR FREE

Kill two birds with one stone by preparing your protein and vegetable in one motion. Green beans provide a host of phytonutrient content, including carotenoids and flavonoids, which all function as anti-inflammatory agents inside the body.

SERVES 4 TO 6

Prep time: 15 minutes or fewer

Cook time: 6 to 7 hours on low

1 pound green beans

1 (2- to 3-pound) whole, boneless turkey breast

2 cups Chimichurri Sauce (page 114; double the recipe)

½ cup broth of choice

1. Put the green beans in the slow cooker. Put the turkey on top. Pour on the sauce and broth.

2. Cover the cooker and set to low. Cook for 6 to 7 hours, or until the internal temperature of the turkey reaches 165°F on a meat thermometer and the juices run clear, and serve.

TIME-SAVING TIP: Don't bother trimming or chopping your green beans. They'll be tender and taste great whole, thanks to the magic of the slow cooker and this chimichurri sauce.

Serving Size: 4 servings
Per Serving: Calories: 776; Total Fat: 59g; Total Carbs: 14g; Sugar: 4g; Fiber: 6g; Protein: 60g; Sodium: 1,128mg

Balsamic-Glazed Turkey Wings

Good-quality balsamic vinegar works to detoxify the body through its antibacterial and anti-inflammatory properties. Like apple cider vinegar, it can bring great relief to stomach upset and digestive troubles. To really caramelize this glaze onto your wings, baste the wings with more of the sauce after removing them from the slow cooker. Put them on a baking sheet and under your oven's preheated broiler for no more than 5 minutes before serving.

SERVES 4 TO 6

Prep time: 15 minutes or fewer

Cook time: 7 to 8 hours on low

1¼ cups balsamic vinegar

2 tablespoons raw honey

1 teaspoon garlic powder

2 pounds turkey wings

1. In a small bowl, whisk the vinegar, honey, and garlic powder.

2. Put the wings in the bottom of the slow cooker, and pour the vinegar sauce on top.

3. Cover the cooker and set to low. Cook for 7 to 8 hours.

4. Baste the wings with the sauce from the bottom of the slow cooker and serve.

INGREDIENT TIP: I didn't include it in the main recipe because it's not a very common ingredient, but arrowroot powder will thicken any sauce that needs some help getting to that perfect texture. Add 1 tablespoon and stir well while the sauce is still hot before spreading it onto the cooked wings.

Serving Size: 4 servings
Per Serving: Calories: 501; Total Fat: 25g; Total Carbs: g; Sugar: 9g; Fiber: 0g; Protein: 47g; Sodium: 162mg

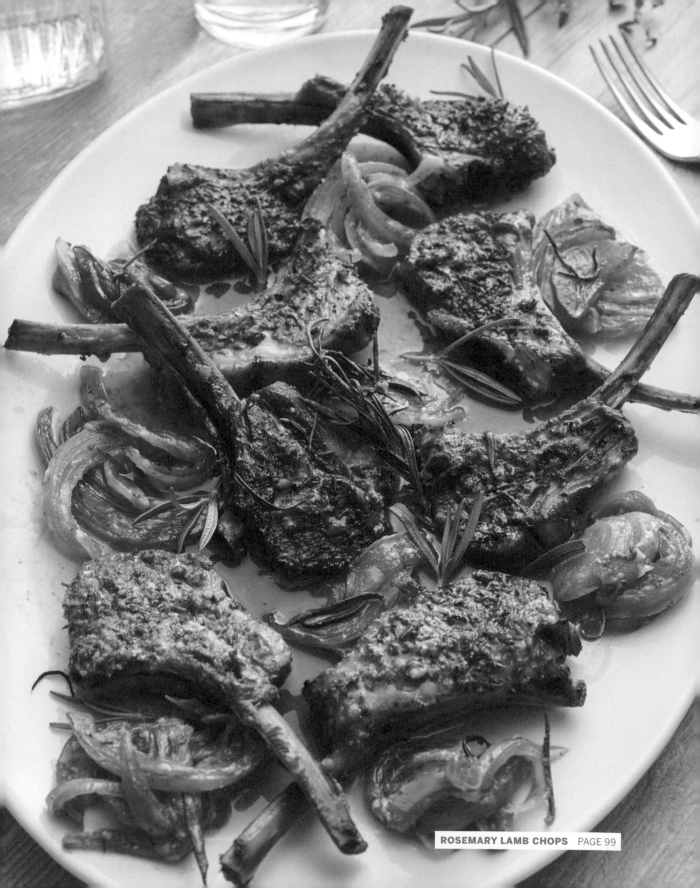

ROSEMARY LAMB CHOPS PAGE 99

6 | MEAT

Beef Bone Broth

CORN FREE | DAIRY FREE | EGG FREE | GLUTEN FREE | NIGHTSHADE FREE | NUT FREE | SOY FREE | SUGAR FREE

Healing and soothing broths like these have been used for centuries the world over, yet they've all but disappeared from American culinary tradition. You don't have to cut corners with your own health! It's soothing to the gut lining and calming to inflammation. If you save your veggie scraps and skins in a freezer bag ahead of time, the slow cooker truly does all the work, and you reap all the benefits. Make sure you get naturally pastured, organic beef marrow bones if possible.

**MAKES ABOUT
4 QUARTS**

Prep time: 15 minutes or fewer

Cook time: 18 to 24 hours on low

2 pounds beef marrow bones

2 cups roughly chopped onions, celery, carrots, garlic, or scraps (a combination based on what's on hand or what you've saved)

2 bay leaves

1 tablespoon apple cider vinegar

Filtered water, to cover the ingredients

1. In your slow cooker, combine the bones, onion, celery, carrots, garlic, bay leaves, and vinegar. Add enough water to cover the ingredients.

2. Cover the cooker and set to low. Cook for 18 to 24 hours. The longer it cooks, the more nutrients you get from the bones and vegetables.

3. Skim off and discard any foam from the surface. Ladle the broth through a fine-mesh sieve or cheesecloth into a large bowl. Transfer to airtight containers to store.

4. Keep refrigerated for 3 to 4 days. Freeze any excess for up to 3 months.

COOKING TIP: If you have extra time, roasting the bones beforehand greatly enhances the flavor of the finished broth. Place the bones in a roasting pan and roast at 400°F for 40 to 60 minutes. Drain off the fat and proceed from the beginning of the recipe.

Serving Size: 1 cup
Per Serving: Calories: 50; Total Fat: 1g; Total Carbs: 2g; Sugar: 0g; Fiber: 0g; Protein: 6g; Sodium: 220mg

Beef & Bell Peppers

CORN FREE | DAIRY FREE | EGG FREE | GLUTEN FREE | NUT FREE | SOY FREE

This Asian-style dish pairs melt-in-your-mouth beef with the inflammatory-fighting power of the capsaicin compounds in colorful bell peppers. They're also rich in quercetin, which produces its own strong anti-inflammatory effect on the body.

SERVES 4 TO 6

Prep time: 15 minutes or fewer

Cook time: 6 to 7 hours on low

1 pound beef tenderloin, cut into 1-inch chunks

1 red bell pepper, seeded and roughly chopped

1 yellow bell pepper, seeded and roughly chopped

1 green bell pepper, seeded and roughly chopped

1 medium onion, chopped

1 (14-ounce) can diced tomatoes

1 cup Beef Bone Broth (page 86) or store-bought broth of choice

¼ cup coconut aminos

1½ teaspoons garlic powder

1 teaspoon coconut sugar

½ teaspoon ground ginger

Dash hot sauce (optional)

Freshly ground black pepper

1. In your slow cooker, combine the beef; red, yellow, and green bell peppers; onion; tomatoes; broth; coconut aminos; garlic powder; coconut sugar; ginger; and hot sauce (if using), and season with black pepper.

2. Cover the cooker and set to low. Cook for 6 to 7 hours and serve.

INGREDIENT TIP: Beef sirloin steak or stewing beef can be used in this recipe instead, as long as the meat is cut into small chunks.

Serving Size: 4 servings

Per Serving: Calories: 411; Total Fat: 10g; Total Carbs: 18g; Sugar: 10g; Fiber: 3g; Protein: 64g; Sodium: 652mg

Korean Beef Lettuce Wraps

CORN FREE | DAIRY FREE | EGG FREE, | GLUTEN FREE | NUT FREE | SOY FREE

By replacing a few ingredients with lighter, anti-inflammatory substitutes, this flavorful dish can be enjoyed without any health qualms. The coconut aminos in this recipe are a soy-free and wheat-free substitute for soy sauce—and taste remarkably similar!

SERVES 4 TO 6

Prep time: 15 minutes or fewer
Cook time: 6 to 7 hours on low

2 pounds beef chuck roast

1 small white onion, diced

1 cup broth of choice

3 tablespoons coconut aminos

2 tablespoons coconut sugar

1 tablespoon rice vinegar

1 teaspoon garlic powder

1 teaspoon sesame oil

½ teaspoon ground ginger

¼ teaspoon red pepper flakes

8 romaine lettuce leaves

1 tablespoon sesame seeds (optional)

2 scallions (both white and green parts), diced (optional)

1. In your slow cooker, combine the beef, onion, broth, coconut aminos, coconut sugar, vinegar, garlic powder, sesame oil, ginger, and red pepper flakes.

2. Cover the cooker and set to low. Cook for 7 to 8 hours.

3. Scoop spoonfuls of the beef mixture into each lettuce leaf. Garnish with sesame seeds and diced scallion (if using) and serve.

INGREDIENT TIP: You can also make this recipe with ground beef, pausing to break it up at the beginning and end of cooking.

Serving Size: 4 servings
Per Serving: Calories: 428; Total Fat: 23g; Total Carbs: 12g; Sugar: 10g; Fiber: 1g; Protein: 46g; Sodium: 425mg

Hearty Bolognese

CORN FREE | DAIRY FREE | EGG FREE | GLUTEN FREE | NUT FREE | SOY FREE | SUGAR FREE

Bolognese traditionally lends itself to hours of hands-on cooking time, stirring frequently over a hot stove, for the flavors to come together. However, a tasty and healthy Bolognese sauce can definitely be made in a slow cooker! The French vegetable trio, *mirepoix* (onion, carrot, and celery), is an anti-inflammatory triple threat with all their antioxidants and flavonoids.

SERVES 4 TO 6

Prep time: 15 minutes or fewer
Cook time: 7 to 8 hours on low

1 tablespoon extra-virgin olive oil

3 garlic cloves, minced

1/2 cup chopped onion

2/3 cup chopped celery

2/3 cup chopped carrot

1 pound ground beef

1 (14-ounce) can diced tomatoes

1 tablespoon white wine vinegar

1/8 teaspoon ground nutmeg

2 bay leaves

1/2 teaspoon red pepper flakes

Dash sea salt

Dash freshly ground black pepper

1. Coat the bottom of the slow cooker with the olive oil.

2. Add the garlic, onion, celery, carrot, ground beef, tomatoes, vinegar, nutmeg, bay leaves, red pepper flakes, salt, and black pepper. Using a fork, break up the ground beef as much as possible.

3. Cover the cooker and set to low. Cook for 7 to 8 hours.

4. Remove and discard the bay leaves. Stir, breaking up the meat completely, and serve.

SERVING TIP: Serve over gluten-free pasta. Aside from brown rice pasta, look for all sorts of wheat pasta substitutes at your grocery store, such as quinoa, lentil, and black bean pasta.

Serving Size: 4 servings
Per Serving: Calories: 314; Total Fat: 21g; Total Carbs: 10g; Sugar: 5g; Fiber: 2g; Protein: 22g; Sodium: 376mg

Herbed Meatballs

CORN FREE | DAIRY FREE | GLUTEN FREE | NUT FREE | SOY FREE | SUGAR FREE

Ground beef can be a wonderfully cost-effective meat to add to an anti-inflammatory diet, as long as it's grass-fed and organic. These two descriptors ensure you get as many healthy omega-3 fatty acids as possible, without any added antibiotics or pesticides to create toxicity in your body. These meatballs are delicious served with Basic Quinoa (page 36), Veggie "Fried" Quinoa (page 41), or Herbed Harvest Rice (page 39).

MAKES 12 MEATBALLS

Prep time: 15 minutes or fewer

Cook time: 7 to 8 hours on low

1½ pounds ground beef

1 large egg

1 small white onion, minced

¼ cup minced mushrooms

1 teaspoon garlic powder

½ teaspoon sea salt

½ teaspoon dried oregano

¼ teaspoon freshly ground black pepper

¼ teaspoon ground ginger

Dash red pepper flakes

1 (14-ounce) can crushed tomatoes

1. In a large bowl, combine the ground beef, egg, onion, mushrooms, garlic powder, salt, oregano, black pepper, ginger, and red pepper flakes. Mix well. Form the beef mixture into about 12 meatballs.

2. Pour the tomatoes into the bottom of your slow cooker. Gently arrange the meatballs on top.

3. Cover the cooker and set to low. Cook for 7 to 8 hours and serve.

COOKING TIP: If you wish to and have the time, to help the meatballs hold their juices, sear them first on a greased baking sheet under your oven's preheated broiler, until browned on each side, before adding to the slow cooker.

Serving Size: 1 meatball
Per Serving: Calories: 131; Total Fat: 8g; Total Carbs: 2g; Sugar: 1g; Fiber: 0g; Protein: 11g; Sodium: 214mg

Pork Ragù

In Italian cooking, ragù is a sauce made from ground meat, onions, and tomato purée and served over pasta. By using a protein-rich gluten-free pasta substitute, such as lentil pasta, you can increase the protein content and get rid of the gluten found in traditional ragù dishes (usually served over pappardelle pasta).

SERVES 4 TO 6

Prep time: 15 minutes or fewer
Cook time: 7 to 8 hours on low

1 pound pork tenderloin

1 medium yellow onion, diced

1 red bell pepper, diced

1 (28-ounce) can diced tomatoes

2 teaspoons chili powder

1 teaspoon garlic powder

½ teaspoon ground cumin

½ teaspoon smoked paprika

Dash red pepper flakes

1 cup fresh spinach leaves, minced

1. In your slow cooker, combine the pork, onion, bell pepper, tomatoes, chili powder, garlic powder, cumin, paprika, red pepper flakes, and spinach.

2. Cover the cooker and set to low. Cook for 7 to 8 hours.

3. Transfer the pork loin to a cutting board and shred with a fork. Return it to the slow cooker, stir it into the sauce, and serve.

COOKING TIP: Like many slow cooker meat recipes, browning or searing the meat for as little as 1 to 3 minutes per side before slow cooking can really seal in flavor in a way that's hard to match.

Serving Size: 4 servings
Per Serving: Calories: 292; Total Fat: 10g; Total Carbs: 15g; Sugar: 8g; Fiber: 3g; Protein: 36g; Sodium: 532mg

Traditional Meatloaf

CORN FREE | DAIRY FREE, | GLUTEN FREE | SOY FREE

Grandma's traditional meatloaf recipe doesn't need to make your health suffer—in fact, I've added some green prowess to it with minced spinach that completely disappears into the yumminess after it's been cooked through.

SERVES 4 TO 6

Prep time: 15 minutes or fewer

Cook time: 5 to 6 hours on low

1 pound lean ground beef

1 small onion, diced

1 cup fresh spinach, minced well

1 large egg, whisked well

½ cup unsweetened almond milk

½ cup all-natural ketchup (choose the one with the lowest amount of sugar)

½ teaspoon sea salt

½ teaspoon garlic powder

½ teaspoon dried sage, minced

½ teaspoon Dijon mustard

1. In your slow cooker, combine the ground beef, onion, spinach, egg, almond milk, ketchup, salt, garlic powder, sage, and mustard. Mix well. Form the meat mixture into a loaf shape, and position it in the center of the slow cooker.

2. Cover the cooker and set to low. Cook for 5 to 6 hours, or until the center of the meatloaf reaches 160°F measured with a meat thermometer, and serve.

INGREDIENT TIP: When choosing nut milks to use in savory meat dishes, be sure to purchase unsweetened and unflavored versions.

Serving Size: 4 servings

Per Serving: Calories: 312; Total Fat: 19g; Total Carbs: 12g; Sugar: 1g; Fiber: 1g; Protein: 23g; Sodium: 747mg

Classic Pot Roast

CORN FREE | DAIRY FREE | EGG FREE | GLUTEN FREE | NIGHTSHADE FREE | NUT FREE | SOY FREE | SUGAR FREE

A warm pot roast is the epitome of comfort food and will fill your home with an enticing, savory aroma. Here I've replaced the usual white potatoes with sweet potatoes for some added beta-carotene, which is an antioxidant helpful in lowering inflammation. Slow cooking this meal until tender presents this often-tough cut of meat in the most easily digested way.

SERVES 6 TO 8

Prep time: 15 minutes or fewer

Cook time: 7 to 8 hours on low

1 teaspoon sea salt

1½ teaspoons dried thyme leaves

1 teaspoon dried rosemary

½ teaspoon freshly ground black pepper

1 (4-pound) beef chuck roast

1 medium onion, sliced

5 carrots, chopped

1 celery stalk, chopped

6 garlic cloves, minced

2 cups broth of choice

3 bay leaves

2 large sweet potatoes, peeled and cubed

1. In a small bowl, stir together the salt, thyme, rosemary, and pepper. Rub the spices all over the roast. Set aside.

2. In your slow cooker, layer the onion, carrots, celery, and garlic on the bottom.

3. Add the broth and bay leaves. Put the meat on top of the vegetables.

4. Put the sweet potatoes on top of the meat.

5. Cover the cooker and set to low. Cook for 7 to 8 hours.

6. Remove and discard the bay leaves before serving.

INGREDIENT TIP: Not everyone enjoys cooking with wine, but know that you can substitute 1 cup of red wine for 1 cup of the broth for added flavor complexity.

Serving Size: 6 servings

Per Serving: Calories: 579; Total Fat: 29g; Total Carbs: 21g; Sugar: 8g; Fiber: 4g; Protein: 63g; Sodium: 660mg

Pulled Pork Tacos

DAIRY FREE | EGG FREE | GLUTEN FREE | NIGHTSHADE FREE | NUT FREE | SOY FREE

In my home we often slow cook a big batch of this pulled pork and freeze half for future easy meals. It's incredibly delicious and versatile. Serve it over rice if you're looking for a corn-free option, or spread the pork onto romaine lettuce leaves for a lettuce wrap.

SERVES 4 TO 6

Prep time: 15 minutes or fewer
Cook time: 7 to 8 hours on low

1 teaspoon sea salt

1 teaspoon ground cumin

1 teaspoon garlic powder

½ teaspoon dried oregano

½ teaspoon freshly ground black pepper

3 to 4 pounds pork shoulder or butt

2 cups broth of choice

Juice of 1 orange

1 small onion, chopped

4 to 6 corn taco shells

Shredded cabbage, lime wedges, avocado, and hot sauce, for topping (optional)

1. In a small bowl, stir together the salt, cumin, garlic powder, oregano, and pepper. Rub the pork with the spice mixture, and put it in your slow cooker.

2. Pour the broth and orange juice around the pork. Scatter the onion around the pork.

3. Cover the cooker and set on low. Cook for 7 to 8 hours.

4. Transfer the pork to a work surface, and shred it with a fork. Serve in taco shells with any optional toppings you like.

INGREDIENT TIP: A great way to make corn more digestible—and its nutrients more full and bioavailable—is to sprout it first. Look for sprouted corn tortillas at your local health food store.

Serving Size: 4 servings

Per Serving: Calories: 1,156; Total Fat: 84g; Total Carbs: 12g; Sugar: 1g; Fiber: 2g; Protein: 84g; Sodium: 942mg

Chili-Lime Pork Loin

Using bright spices, tangy citrus juices, and rich broths are favorite ways of mine to create recipes bursting with flavor without sacrificing their nutrient integrity. Each of these entities works with your body to lower inflammation and nourish it, as opposed to so many store-bought sauces and gravies that weigh us down and have a long list of health-busting preservatives.

SERVES 4 TO 6

Prep time: 15 minutes or fewer

Cook time: 6 to 7 hours on low

3 teaspoons chili powder

2 teaspoons garlic powder

1 teaspoon ground cumin

½ teaspoon sea salt

2 (1-pound) pork tenderloins

1 cup broth of choice

¼ cup freshly squeezed lime juice

1. In a small bowl, stir together the chili powder, garlic powder, cumin, and salt. Rub the pork all over with the spice mixture, and put it in the slow cooker.

2. Pour the broth and lime juice around the pork in the cooker.

3. Cover the cooker and set to low. Cook for 6 to 7 hours.

4. Remove the pork from the slow cooker and let rest for 5 minutes. Slice the pork against the grain into medallions before serving.

COOKING TIP: I've found that marinating meats for lengthy periods of time before cooking isn't as necessary with a slow cooker because, in the slow cooker, the meat gets plenty of time to mingle with the other flavors.

Serving Size: 4 servings

Per Serving: Calories: 259; Total Fat: 5g; Total Carbs: 5g; Sugar: 0g; Fiber: 1g; Protein: 50g; Sodium: 510mg

Sausage & White Bean Soup

CORN FREE | DAIRY FREE | EGG FREE | GLUTEN FREE | NIGHTSHADE FREE | NUT FREE | SOY FREE | SUGAR FREE

Bay leaves are used throughout this cookbook, but have you ever wondered why? They heavily aid the digestibility of the food they are cooked with. Bay leaves also contain parthenolide, a compound that—when used topically or ingested regularly—works to greatly reduce inflammation in the body, like that associated with arthritis.

SERVES 4 TO 6

Prep time: 15 minutes or fewer
Cook time: 6 to 7 hours on low

1 pound pre-cooked pork sausage, thinly sliced into coins

2 (15-ounce) cans cannellini beans, rinsed and drained well

5 carrots, diced

1 medium onion, diced

1 celery stalk, minced

2 bay leaves

1 teaspoon garlic powder

½ teaspoon dried oregano

½ teaspoon dried basil leaves

6 cups broth of choice

4 cups shredded, de-ribbed kale

1. In your slow cooker, combine the sausage, beans, carrots, onion, celery, bay leaves, garlic powder, oregano, basil, broth, and kale.

2. Cover the cooker and set to low. Cook for 6 to 7 hours.

3. Remove and discard the bay leaves before serving.

TIME-SAVING TIP: Look for prepackaged bags of torn kale that already have the ribs removed at the grocery store.

Serving Size: 4 servings
Per Serving: Calories: 712; Total Fat: 36g; Total Carbs: 52g; Sugar: 9g; Fiber: 13g; Protein: 47g; Sodium: 1,926mg

Lamb Meatballs with Dill Sauce

CORN FREE | DAIRY FREE | GLUTEN FREE | NUT FREE | SOY FREE | SUGAR FREE

These meatballs have a beautiful Mediterranean vibe to them, and the unique combination of spices and herbs only adds to their anti-inflammatory power. Pumpkin pie spice may seem like an odd addition to a savory dish, but it contains great proportions of ginger, cinnamon, nutmeg, and allspice, which allows you to measure only once.

MAKES 12 MEATBALLS

Prep time: 15 minutes or fewer
Cook time: 7 to 8 hours on low

1½ pounds ground lamb

1 small white onion, minced

1 large egg

1 teaspoon garlic powder

½ teaspoon sea salt

½ teaspoon ground cumin

½ teaspoon pumpkin
pie spice

½ teaspoon paprika

¼ teaspoon freshly ground
black pepper

1 cup Avocado-Dill Sauce
(page 117)

1. In a large bowl, combine the lamb, onion, egg, garlic powder, salt, cumin, pumpkin pie spice, paprika, and pepper. Mix well. Form the lamb mixture into about 12 meatballs. Arrange the meatballs along the bottom of your slow cooker.

2. Cover the cooker and set on low. Cook for 7 to 8 hours.

3. Serve with the avocado-dill sauce.

SERVING TIP: While pasta and rice are common accompaniments when serving meatballs, try these cooled on top of a bed of mixed greens for a Mediterranean meatball salad.

Serving Size: 1 meatball
Per Serving: Calories: 200; Total Fat: 17g; Total Carbs: 2g; Sugar: 0g; Fiber: 1g; Protein: 10g; Sodium: 138mg

Roasted Leg of Lamb

CORN FREE | DAIRY FREE | EGG FREE | GLUTEN FREE | NIGHTSHADE FREE | NUT FREE | SOY FREE | SUGAR FREE

If you're choosing grass-fed organic lamb, this meat can be a great addition to an anti-inflammatory diet. These specific animals have been shown to have more anti-inflammatory omega-3 fatty acids and fewer pro-inflammatory omega-6 fatty acids than corn-fed animals.

SERVES 4 TO 6

Prep time: 15 minutes or fewer

Cook time: 5 to 6 hours on low

1½ teaspoons sea salt

½ teaspoon freshly ground black pepper

1 teaspoon garlic powder

1 teaspoon dried thyme leaves

1 teaspoon dried rosemary

1 teaspoons Dijon mustard

1 (4-pound) bone-in lamb leg

2 cups broth of choice

1 small onion, roughly chopped

1. In a small bowl, stir together the salt, pepper, garlic powder, thyme, rosemary, and mustard to make a paste. Rub the paste evenly onto the lamb, and put it in the slow cooker.

2. Add the broth and onion around the lamb in the cooker.

3. Cover the cooker and set to low. Cook for 5 to 6 hours and serve.

INGREDIENT TIP: Be sure to get a leg of lamb that fits into the shape and size of your slow cooker. If you own a circular slow cooker, rather than oval, you may need to have your butcher cut it in half.

Serving Size: 4 servings
Per Serving: Calories: 780; Total Fat: 41g; Total Carbs: 3g; Sugar: 1g; Fiber: 0g; Protein: 93g; Sodium: 1,023mg

Rosemary Lamb Chops

CORN FREE | DAIRY FREE | EGG FREE | GLUTEN FREE | NIGHTSHADE FREE | NUT FREE | SOY FREE | SUGAR FREE

In addition to omega-3s, lamb contains another beneficial fatty acid called conjugated linoleic acid (CLA). In grass-fed lamb, this fatty acid has been associated with reduced inflammation. Grass-fed lamb is also high in the antioxidants zinc and selenium, which protect against inflammation-causing oxidative stress in the body.

SERVES 4 TO 6

Prep time: 15 minutes or fewer

Cook time: 7 to 8 hours on low

1 medium onion, sliced

2 teaspoons garlic powder

2 teaspoons dried rosemary

1 teaspoon sea salt

½ teaspoon dried
thyme leaves

Freshly ground black pepper

8 bone-in lamb chops (about
3 pounds)

2 tablespoons
balsamic vinegar

1. Line the bottom of the slow cooker with the onion slices.

2. In a small bowl, stir together the garlic powder, rosemary, salt, thyme, and pepper. Rub the chops evenly with the spice mixture, and gently place them in the slow cooker.

3. Drizzle the vinegar over the top.

4. Cover the cooker and set to low. Cook for 7 to 8 hours and serve.

COOKING TIP: Extra liquid isn't necessary here because the juice from the cooking lamb chops provides enough moisture.

Serving Size: 4 servings

Per Serving: Calories: 327; Total Fat: 14g; Total Carbs: 4g; Sugar: 1g; Fiber: 1g; Protein: 43g; Sodium: 1,170mg

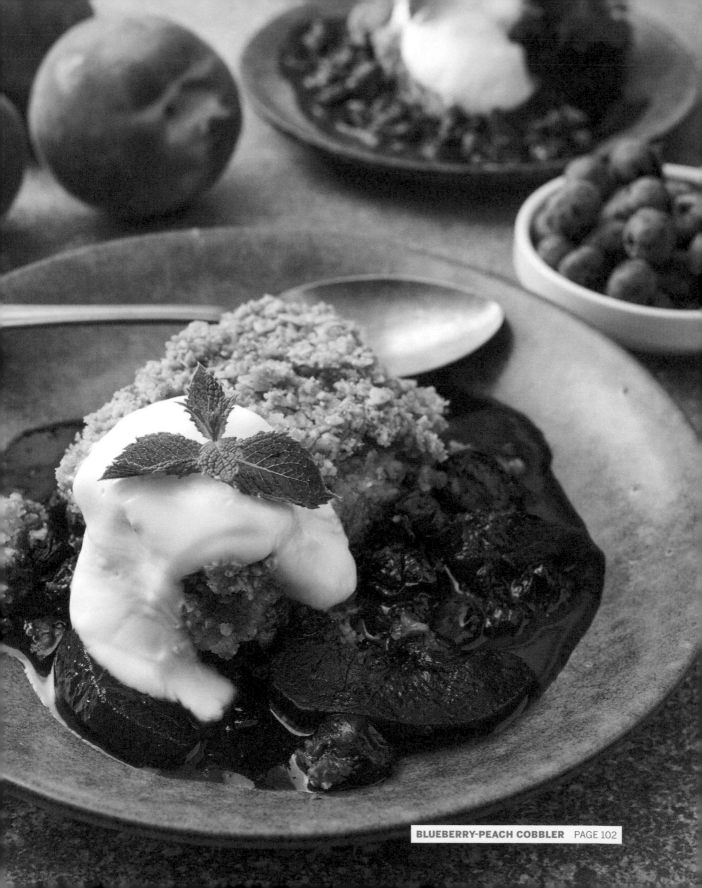

BLUEBERRY-PEACH COBBLER PAGE 102

7 | DESSERT

Blueberry-Peach Cobbler

CORN FREE | DAIRY FREE | EGG FREE | GLUTEN FREE | NIGHTSHADE FREE | SOY FREE | VEGAN

This version of a sweet comfort food helps keep inflammation in check by *omitting* certain highly reactive ingredients, such as all-purpose wheat flour, refined white sugar, and unhealthy fats, but still including sweet, indulgent flavors. Enjoy this dessert with a scoop of Coconut-Vanilla Yogurt (page 107).

SERVES 4 TO 6

Prep time: 15 minutes or fewer

Cook time: 2 hours on high

5 tablespoons coconut oil, divided

3 large peaches, peeled and sliced

2 cups frozen blueberries

1 cup almond flour

1 cup rolled oats

1 tablespoon maple syrup

1 tablespoon coconut sugar

1 teaspoon ground cinnamon

½ teaspoon vanilla extract

Pinch ground nutmeg

1. Coat the bottom of your slow cooker with 1 tablespoon of coconut oil.

2. Arrange the peaches and blueberries along the bottom of the slow cooker.

3. In a small bowl, stir together the almond flour, oats, remaining 4 tablespoons of coconut oil, maple syrup, coconut sugar, cinnamon, vanilla, and nutmeg until a coarse mixture forms. Gently crumble the topping over the fruit in the slow cooker.

4. Cover the cooker and set to high. Cook for 2 hours and serve.

COOKING TIP: You can help keep the top "crust" of the cobbler crisp by placing a paper towel over the slow cooker opening before putting the lid on securely. This helps soak up extra moisture.

Serving Size: 4 servings

Per Serving: Calories: 516; Total Fat: 34g; Total Carbs: 49g; Sugar: 24g; Fiber: 10g; Protein: 10g; Sodium: 1mg

Chai Spice Baked Apples

CORN FREE | DAIRY FREE | EGG FREE | GLUTEN FREE | NIGHTSHADE FREE | SOY FREE | SUGAR FREE | VEGAN

Cloves, ginger, and cinnamon are the base spices in a good chai blend, but they may also help eliminate pain associated with inflammation and arthritis. Ginger specifically has properties similar to ibuprofen.

MAKES 5 APPLES

Prep time: 15 minutes or fewer
Cook time: 2 to 3 hours on high

5 apples

½ cup water

½ cup crushed pecans (optional)

¼ cup melted coconut oil

1 teaspoon ground cinnamon

½ teaspoon ground ginger

¼ teaspoon ground cardamom

¼ teaspoon ground cloves

1. Core each apple, and peel off a thin strip from the top of each.

2. Add the water to the slow cooker. Gently place each apple upright along the bottom.

3. In a small bowl, stir together the pecans (if using), coconut oil, cinnamon, ginger, cardamom, and cloves. Drizzle the mixture over the tops of the apples.

4. Cover the cooker and set to high. Cook for 2 to 3 hours, until the apples soften, and serve.

INGREDIENT TIP: Try stuffing the finished baked apples with Coconut-Vanilla Yogurt (page 107) or Sour Cherry & Pumpkin Seed Granola (page 22).

Serving Size: 1 apple
Per Serving: Calories: 217; Total Fat: 12g; Total Carbs: 30g; Sugar: 22g; Fiber: 6g; Protein: 0g; Sodium: 0mg

Cacao Brownies

CORN FREE | DAIRY FREE | GLUTEN FREE | NIGHTSHADE FREE | SOY FREE

The almond butter in this recipe replaces the dairy butter you usually find in brownies. Nuts such as almonds have an anti-inflammatory effect because they contain high amounts of vitamin E, which protects the body against free radicals.

SERVES 4 TO 6

Prep time: 15 minutes or fewer
Cook time: 2½ to 3 hours on low

3 tablespoons coconut oil, divided

1 cup almond butter

1 cup unsweetened cacao powder

½ cup coconut sugar

2 large eggs

2 ripe bananas

2 teaspoons vanilla extract

1 teaspoon baking soda

½ teaspoon sea salt

1. Coat the bottom of the slow cooker with 1 tablespoon of coconut oil.

2. In a medium bowl, combine the almond butter, cacao powder, coconut sugar, eggs, bananas, vanilla, baking soda, and salt. Mash the bananas and stir well until a batter forms. Pour the batter into the slow cooker.

3. Cover the cooker and set to low. Cook for 2½ to 3 hours, until firm to a light touch but still gooey in the middle, and serve.

SERVING TIP: Using an electric handheld mixer, you can whip ½ cup of coconut cream into a thick and fluffy frosting to go on top if you want to add some healthy fats and flavor.

Serving Size: 4 servings
Per Serving: Calories: 779; Total Fat: 51g; Total Carbs: 68g; Sugar: 35g; Fiber: 15g; Protein: 18g; Sodium: 665mg

Cinnamon Pecans

CORN FREE | DAIRY FREE | GLUTEN FREE | NIGHTSHADE FREE | SOY FREE

When living an anti-inflammatory lifestyle, it's important to choose sweeteners that are whole, real foods, not stripped of the minerals they possess. Both maple syrup and coconut sugar contain trace amounts of magnesium, phosphorus, calcium, and potassium. While neither is a superfood, each adds more value than refined white sugar does.

MAKES ABOUT 3½ CUPS

Prep time: 15 minutes or fewer

Cook time: 3 to 4 hours on low

1 tablespoon coconut oil

1 large egg white

2 tablespoons ground cinnamon

2 teaspoons vanilla extract

¼ cup maple syrup

2 tablespoons coconut sugar

¼ teaspoon sea salt

3 cups pecan halves

1. Coat the slow cooker with the coconut oil.

2. In a medium bowl, whisk the egg white.

3. Add the cinnamon, vanilla, maple syrup, coconut sugar, and salt. Whisk well to combine.

4. Add the pecans and stir to coat. Pour the pecans into the slow cooker.

5. Cover the cooker and set to low. Cook for 3 to 4 hours.

6. Remove the pecans from the slow cooker and spread them on a baking sheet or other cooling surface. Let cool for 5 to 10 minutes before serving. Store in an airtight container at room temperature for up to 2 weeks.

COOKING TIP: If you're nearby your slow cooker, give your pecans a good stir halfway through the cooking time to break up any chunks in the coating.

Serving Size: ¼ cup
Per Serving: Calories: 195; Total Fat: 18g; Total Carbs: 9g; Sugar: 6g; Fiber: 3g; Protein: 2g; Sodium: 46mg

Missouri Haystack Cookies

CORN FREE | DAIRY FREE | EGG FREE | GLUTEN FREE | NIGHTSHADE FREE | SOY FREE | VEGAN

Replacing a cup of sugar with an overripe banana provides sweetness without all the inflammation-causing refined white sugar. The riper the banana, the more time it's had to convert its complex carbohydrates to simple sugar, and the taste speaks for itself!

MAKES ABOUT 24 SMALL COOKIES

Prep time: 15 minutes or fewer

Cook time: 1½ hours on high

½ cup coconut oil

½ cup unsweetened almond milk

1 overripe banana, mashed well

½ cup coconut sugar

¼ cup cacao powder

1 teaspoon vanilla extract

¼ teaspoon sea salt

3 cups rolled oats

½ cup almond butter

1. In a medium bowl, stir together the coconut oil, almond milk, mashed banana, coconut sugar, cacao powder, vanilla, and salt. Pour the mixture into the slow cooker.

2. Pour the oats on top without stirring.

3. Put the almond butter on top of the oats without stirring.

4. Cover the cooker and set to high. Cook for 1½ hours.

5. Stir the mixture well. As it cools, scoop tablespoon-size balls out and press onto a baking sheet to continue to cool. Serve when hardened. Keep leftovers refrigerated in an airtight container for up to 1 week.

INGREDIENT TIP: For added texture, use crunchy nut butter.

Serving Size: 1 cookie

Per Serving: Calories: 140; Total Fat: 9g; Total Carbs: 14g; Sugar: 5g; Fiber: 2g; Protein: 2g; Sodium: 29mg

Coconut-Vanilla Yogurt

Once you get comfortable with this amazing dairy-free yogurt recipe, you can begin to experiment with the ingredient ratios to make it thicker or thinner to suit your preferences. The probiotics in this tangy treat may help reduce certain biomarkers of inflammation in the body, such as C-reactive protein, which helps protect against such conditions as cardiovascular disease and cancer. Getting the temperature right is important, so you'll need a candy thermometer.

MAKES ABOUT 3½ CUPS

Prep time: 15 minutes or fewer
Cook time: 1 to 2 hours on high, plus overnight to ferment

3 (13.5-ounce) cans full-fat coconut milk

5 probiotic capsules (not pills)

1 teaspoon raw honey

½ teaspoon vanilla extract

1. Pour the coconut milk into the slow cooker.

2. Cover the cooker and set to high. Cook for 1 to 2 hours, until the temperature of the milk reaches 180°F measured with a candy thermometer.

3. Turn off the slow cooker and allow the temperature of the milk to come down close to 100°F.

4. Open the probiotic capsules and pour in the contents, along with the honey and vanilla. Stir well to combine.

5. Re-cover the slow cooker, turn it off and unplug it, and wrap it in an insulating towel to keep warm overnight as it ferments.

6. Pour the yogurt into sterilized jars and refrigerate. The yogurt should thicken slightly in the refrigerator, where it will keep for up to 1 week.

COOKING TIP: The finished product should taste tangy, even amidst the vanilla flavor. Throw it away if it tastes spoiled—sometimes cultured foods can have a mind of their own even when you follow the directions!

Serving Size: ½ cup
Per Serving: Calories: 305; Total Fat: 30g; Total Carbs: 7g; Sugar: 3g; Fiber: 0g; Protein: 2g; Sodium: 43mg

Salted Dark Drinking Chocolate

CORN FREE | DAIRY FREE | EGG FREE | GLUTEN FREE | NIGHTSHADE FREE | SOY FREE

The flavanols (phytonutrient compounds with an antioxidant effect) in cacao may reduce or even prevent inflammation of the blood vessels, or vascular inflammation. When vascular inflammation is lowered, circulation should improve, as should any previous cramping or pain in the limbs.

MAKES 4 TO 6 CUPS

Prep time: 15 minutes or fewer
Cook time: 3 to 4 hours on low

5 cups unsweetened
almond milk

2½ tablespoons coconut oil

5 tablespoons cacao powder

5 cinnamon sticks

3 to 4 teaspoons coconut
sugar or raw honey

1 tablespoon vanilla extract

1 (3-inch) piece fresh ginger

1 (2-inch) piece turmeric root

3 tablespoons collagen
peptides

½ to ¾ teaspoon sea
salt, divided

1. In your slow cooker, combine the almond milk, coconut oil, cacao powder, cinnamon sticks, coconut sugar or honey, vanilla, ginger, and turmeric.

2. Cover the cooker and set to low. Cook for 3 to 4 hours.

3. Pour the contents of the cooker through a fine-mesh sieve into a clean container; discard the solids.

4. Stir in the collagen peptides until well combined.

5. Pour the chocolate into mugs and gently sprinkle ⅛ teaspoon of sea salt on top of each beverage. Serve hot.

INGREDIENT TIP: The collagen peptides act as a perfect protein source to balance out this sweet beverage and keep your blood sugar levels balanced, therefore holding inflammation in check! Plus, collagen peptides are tasteless, so you won't notice them at all.

Serving Size: 4 servings
Per Serving: Calories: 235; Total Fat: 14g; Total Carbs: 20g; Sugar: 12g; Fiber: 4g; Protein: 7g; Sodium: 512mg

Warm Cinnamon-Turmeric Almond Milk

CORN FREE | DAIRY FREE | EGG FREE | GLUTEN FREE | NIGHTSHADE FREE | SOY FREE

Turmeric is arguably the one herb you want to make sure you add into your anti-inflammatory diet at all cost. It is known as a natural pain reliever, a wound healer, and a liver protector. Curcumin, the popular compound in turmeric, has anti-inflammatory powers that have been shown to be as effective as many anti-inflammatory drugs (including cortisone), but without the ugly side effects.

MAKES 4 TO 6 CUPS

Prep time: 15 minutes or fewer

Cook time: 3 to 4 hours on low

4 cups unsweetened almond milk

4 cinnamon sticks

2 tablespoons coconut oil

1 (4-inch) piece turmeric root, roughly chopped

1 (2-inch) piece fresh ginger, roughly chopped

1 teaspoon raw honey, plus more to taste

1. In your slow cooker, combine the almond milk, cinnamon sticks, coconut oil, turmeric, and ginger.

2. Cover the cooker and set to low. Cook for 3 to 4 hours.

3. Pour the contents of the cooker through a fine-mesh sieve into a clean container; discard the solids.

4. Starting with just 1 teaspoon, add raw honey to taste.

INGREDIENT TIP: Black pepper aids in the absorption of curcumin, so add a few pinches to this beverage if you aren't allergic.

Serving Size: 4 servings

Per Serving: Calories: 133; Total Fat: 11g; Total Carbs: 10g; Sugar: 7g; Fiber: 1g; Protein: 1g; Sodium: 152mg

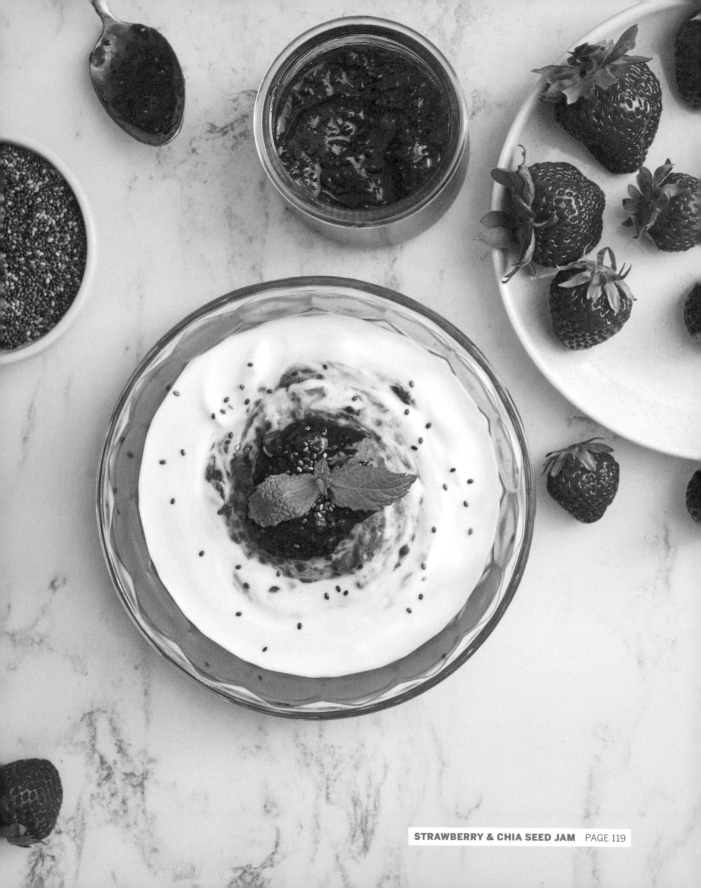

STRAWBERRY & CHIA SEED JAM PAGE 119

8 | SAUCES & STAPLES

Garden Marinara Sauce

CORN FREE | DAIRY FREE | EGG FREE | GLUTEN FREE | NUT FREE | SOY FREE | SUGAR FREE | VEGAN

My goal with this cookbook is to give you easy recipes using on-hand pantry items. However, this particular recipe would be a fantastic place to incorporate fresh herbs, as they are even more potent in their anti-inflammatory powers than dried. Simply triple the amount of herbs called for in this recipe if using fresh.

MAKES ABOUT 6 CUPS

Prep time: 15 minutes or fewer

Cook time: 7 to 8 hours on low

2 (28-ounce) cans diced tomatoes

3 tablespoons tomato paste

1 yellow onion, diced

1 carrot, minced

1 celery stalk, minced

2 bay leaves

1 tablespoon dried basil leaves

2 teaspoons dried oregano

1½ teaspoons garlic powder

1 teaspoon sea salt

Pinch red pepper flakes

Freshly ground black pepper

1. In your slow cooker, combine the tomatoes, tomato paste, onion, carrot, celery, bay leaves, basil, oregano, garlic powder, salt, and red pepper flakes, and season with black pepper.

2. Cover the cooker and set it to low. Cook for 7 to 8 hours.

3. Remove and discard the bay leaves. Using an immersion blender, blend the sauce to your desired consistency, or leave it naturally chunky.

MAKE-AHEAD TIP: This sauce easily freezes for up to 3 months. Just cool it completely before putting into freezer-safe containers.

Serving Size: 1 cup
Per Serving: Calories: 71; Total Fat: 0g; Total Carbs: 17g; Sugar: 11g; Fiber: 3g; Protein: 3g; Sodium: 1,091mg

Tangy Barbecue Sauce with Apple Cider Vinegar

CORN FREE | DAIRY FREE | EGG FREE | NUT FREE

This recipe cuts way down on those added (inflammatory) sweeteners compared to store-bought barbecue sauces. There is also plenty of room to spice it up or tone it down with sweetness by experimenting with the cayenne and other whole-food sweetener options.

MAKES ABOUT 2 CUPS

Prep time: 15 minutes or fewer

Cook time: 3 to 4 hours on low

1¼ cups all-natural ketchup (choose the one with the lowest amount of sugar)

¼ cup molasses

¼ cup coconut sugar

3 tablespoons apple cider vinegar

1 tablespoon Worcestershire sauce

1½ teaspoons garlic powder

1 teaspoon Dijon mustard

½ teaspoon sea salt

½ teaspoon onion powder

Pinch cayenne pepper

1. In your slow cooker, combine the ketchup, molasses, coconut sugar, vinegar, Worcestershire sauce, garlic powder, mustard, salt, onion powder, and cayenne.

2. Cover the cooker and set it to low. Cook for 3 to 4 hours.

3. Let cool and refrigerate in an airtight container.

MAKE-AHEAD TIP: This sauce will keep refrigerated in an airtight container for up to 1 week.

Serving Size: 1 cup
Per Serving: Calories: 416; Total Fat: 0g; Total Carbs: 105g; Sugar: 95g; Fiber: 0g; Protein: 0g; Sodium: 2,649mg

Chimichurri Sauce

Here's an easy way to add flavor without your slow cooker. All you need in terms of appliances is a high-speed blender, food processor, or immersion blender—take your pick! Parsley is the main ingredient here, and while it's a rather underrated ingredient, it contains apigenin, a flavonoid that shakes inflammation to its core.

MAKES ABOUT 1 CUP

Prep time: 15 minutes or fewer

1 cup fresh flat-leaf Italian parsley

½ cup fresh cilantro

½ cup extra-virgin olive oil

¼ cup white wine vinegar

3 garlic cloves, roughly chopped

½ teaspoon sea salt

½ teaspoon dried oregano

¼ teaspoon ground cumin

Dash red pepper flakes

Freshly ground black pepper

In a blender, food processor, or large bowl, combine the parsley, cilantro, olive oil, vinegar, garlic, salt, oregano, cumin, and red pepper flakes, and season with black pepper. Blend until smooth. Serve at room temperature as part of the Chimichurri Turkey & Green Beans (page 82). It is also great over red meat dishes. Refrigerate any leftovers in an airtight container for up to 1 week.

STORAGE TIP: You can freeze portions of chimichurri in ice cube trays and easily pop out one at a time to thaw as needed.

Serving Size: 1 recipe
Per Serving: Calories: 1,018; Total Fat: 112g; Total Carbs: 14g; Sugar: 1g; Fiber: 5g; Protein: 4g; Sodium: 1,198mg

Caramelized Onions

CORN FREE | DAIRY FREE | EGG FREE | GLUTEN FREE | NIGHTSHADE FREE | NUT FREE | SOY FREE | SUGAR FREE | VEGAN

There is a lot of science behind caramelizing onions, but you don't have to overcomplicate the process! Just know that you do not have to add pro-inflammatory white sugar to end up with sweet onions, and you also need to start with way more onions than you think you'll need. This recipe makes about 2 cups, but you can essentially fill your slow cooker three-quarters full, depending on its size, to make more—the onions shrink to roughly a quarter of their original volume.

MAKES ABOUT 2 CUPS

Prep time: 15 minutes or fewer

Cook time: 10 hours on low

4 large onions (white or sweet), sliced very thin

2 tablespoons extra-virgin olive oil

½ teaspoon sea salt

1. In your slow cooker, combine the onions, olive oil, and salt. Stir to coat the onions with the oil.

2. Cover the cooker and set it to low. Cook for 10 hours. Drain the liquid and serve.

MAKE-AHEAD TIP: These onions freeze nicely in airtight freezer containers for up to 3 months. To thaw, move to the refrigerator the day before you need them, or run the container under warm water until thawed.

Serving Size: 1 cup
Per Serving: Calories: 234. Total Fat: 14g; Total Carbs: 26g; Sugar: 13g; Fiber: 5g; Protein: 3g; Sodium: 590mg

Vegan Buffalo Dip

CORN FREE | DAIRY FREE | EGG FREE | GLUTEN FREE | SOY FREE | SUGAR FREE | VEGAN

Buffalo dip is typically packed with inflammatory processed cheeses and preservatives. Not here—but don't let all the veggies deter you. Steamed cauliflower and soaked cashews are favorites in the vegan community for thickening sauces and dips, with a neutral flavor and antioxidants to boot.

SERVES 4 TO 6

Prep time: 15 minutes, plus 8 hours to soak

Cook time: 5 to 6 hours on low

1 pound cauliflower, chopped

1¼ cups raw cashews, soaked in water overnight, drained

¾ cup hot sauce (see Tip)

½ cup water

1 tablespoon freshly squeezed lemon juice

1 teaspoon garlic powder

½ teaspoon paprika

Sea salt

Freshly ground black pepper

Chopped veggies, for serving (optional)

1. In your slow cooker, combine the cauliflower, cashews, hot sauce, water, lemon juice, garlic powder, and paprika. Season with salt and pepper.

2. Cover the cooker and set to low. Cook for 5 to 6 hours.

3. Transfer the mixture to a blender or food processor. Pulse until the desired consistency is reached. Serve with chopped veggies (if using).

INGREDIENT TIP: Frank's RedHot Original Cayenne Pepper Sauce has ingredients this cookbook approves of.

Serving Size: 4 servings
Per Serving: Calories: 302; Total Fat: 18g; Total Carbs: 26g; Sugar: 14g; Fiber: 6g; Protein: 9g; Sodium: 574mg

Avocado-Dill Sauce

CORN FREE | DAIRY FREE | EGG FREE | GLUTEN FREE | NUT FREE | SOY FREE | SUGAR FREE | VEGAN

This creamy dipping sauce combines several inflammation-fighting foods. Avocados are known for soothing inflammation through their rich fiber and many antioxidants, such as vitamins E and C and the mineral manganese. And dill, while not the most popular kitchen herb, has been shown to possess powerful analgesic and anti-inflammatory properties.

MAKES ABOUT 1 CUP

Prep time: 15 minutes or fewer

1 large, ripe avocado, peeled and pitted

2 teaspoons fresh dill

2 teaspoons freshly squeezed lemon juice

½ teaspoon sea salt

Dash red pepper flakes

Chopped veggies, for serving (if desired)

In a blender, combine the avocado, dill, lemon juice, salt, and red pepper flakes. Pulse until smooth. If the sauce is too thick, add water to thin as needed. Serve with chopped veggies (if using).

PREPARATION TIP: If you don't have a high-speed blender, put the ingredients in a tall jar and use an immersion blender to make the sauce.

Serving Size. 1 recipe
Per Serving: Calories: 301; Total Fat: 27g; Total Carbs: 19g; Sugar: 2g; Fiber: 12g; Protein: 4g; Sodium: 1,177mg

Creamy Turmeric Dressing

CORN FREE | DAIRY FREE | EGG FREE | GLUTEN FREE | NIGHTSHADE FREE | NUT FREE | SOY FREE

Too many store-bought salad dressings and marinades contain pro-inflammatory oils, such as canola or soybean, as their main ingredient. By making a simple dressing for the week at home, you avoid potentially oxidized fats and can customize it by adding additional anti-inflammatory ingredients, such as turmeric.

SERVES 4 TO 6

Prep time: 15 minutes or fewer

¼ cup extra-virgin olive oil

2 tablespoons water

2 tablespoons freshly squeezed lemon juice

1½ tablespoons raw honey

1 tablespoon apple cider vinegar

1 teaspoon ground turmeric

1 teaspoon Dijon mustard

½ teaspoon ground ginger

¼ teaspoon sea salt

Pinch freshly ground black pepper

In a small bowl, combine the olive oil, water, lemon juice, honey, vinegar, turmeric, mustard, ginger, salt, and pepper. Whisk well to combine. Keep refrigerated in an airtight container.

STORAGE TIP: You can easily double this recipe. It will keep, refrigerated in an airtight container, for up to 1 week.

Serving Size: 4 servings
Per Serving: Calories: 151; Total Fat: 14g; Total Carbs: 8g; Sugar: 7g; Fiber: 0g; Protein: 0g; Sodium: 176mg

Strawberry & Chia Seed Jam

CORN FREE | DAIRY FREE | EGG FREE | GLUTEN FREE | NIGHTSHADE FREE | NUT FREE | SOY FREE

Chia seeds come from a flowering plant in the mint family that's native to Mexico and Guatemala. They may be tiny, but they're powerfully loaded with omega-3 fats, protein, dietary fiber, and antioxidants. And they absorb water, helping you feel full and satiated after eating them.

MAKES ABOUT 2½ CUPS

Prep time: 15 minutes or fewer

Cook time: 3 to 4 hours on high

2 cups strawberries, fresh or frozen, stemmed and quartered

1 cup water

2 tablespoons chia seeds

2 tablespoons raw honey, or to taste (optional)

2 teaspoons freshly squeezed lemon juice

1. In your the slow cooker, combine the strawberries, water, chia seeds, honey (if using), and lemon juice.

2. Cover the cooker and set to high. Cook for 3 to 4 hours.

3. Remove the lid and mash with a potato masher or fork. If you prefer a smooth jam without any visible seeds, use an immersion blender after the jam cools. Refrigerate in an airtight container.

INGREDIENT TIP: You can use chia jam to replace eggs in many sweet recipes, such as strawberry pancakes, by replacing each egg called for with 3 tablespoons chia jam.

Serving Size: 2½ tablespoons

Per Serving: Calories: 14; Total Fat: 0g; Total Carbs: 5g; Sugar: 1g; Fiber: 1g; Protein: 0.5g; Sodium: 0mg

Old-Fashioned Applesauce

CORN FREE | DAIRY FREE | EGG FREE | GLUTEN FREE | NIGHTSHADE FREE | NUT FREE | SOY FREE | SUGAR FREE | VEGAN

Apples are high in polyphenols, a protective compound found in many plants that may protect against inflammation. Enjoy this comforting and naturally sweet treat, warm or chilled, any time of day.

SERVES 4 TO 6

Prep time: 15 minutes or fewer

Cook time: 6 to 8 hours on low

3 pounds apples of choice, peeled, cored, and roughly chopped

½ cup water

1 teaspoon freshly squeezed lemon juice

½ teaspoon pumpkin pie spice

1. In your slow cooker, combine the apples, water, lemon juice, and pumpkin pie spice.

2. Cover the cooker and set to low. Cook for 6 to 8 hours. If you prefer a smoother applesauce, use an immersion blender after the applesauce cools. Refrigerate in an airtight container.

INGREDIENT TIP: Don't be afraid to use slightly older or mealy apples in this recipe. Once they are cooked down, you'll never notice the difference!

Serving Size: 4 servings
Per Serving: Calories: 181; Total Fat: 1g; Total Carbs: 48g; Sugar: 36g; Fiber: 8g; Protein: 1g; Sodium: 0mg

Vanilla-Pear Butter

CORN FREE | DAIRY FREE | EGG FREE | GLUTEN FREE | NIGHTSHADE FREE | NUT FREE | SOY FREE | VEGAN

Much of a pear's natural antioxidant and phytonutrient content is found in the peel, so don't peel them before cooking! They are also rich in the antioxidant vitamin C and boast almost a quarter of your daily fiber content. Taste the pear butter before adding any coconut sugar—you may find it plenty sweet on its own!

MAKES ABOUT 3 CUPS

Prep time: 15 minutes or fewer
Cook time: 6 to 8 hours on low

3 pounds unpeeled pears, cored and cut into chunks

½ cup water

1 tablespoon freshly squeezed lemon juice

2 teaspoons ground cinnamon

1 teaspoon vanilla extract

½ teaspoon ground ginger

1½ teaspoons coconut sugar (optional)

1. In your slow cooker, combine the pears, water, lemon juice, cinnamon, vanilla, and ginger.

2. Cover the cooker and set to low. Cook for 6 to 8 hours. Transfer to a blender or food processor and purée until smooth.

3. Taste and add coconut sugar as needed. Refrigerate in an airtight container.

STORAGE TIP: You can easily freeze extra pear butter in zip-top freezer bags for up to 3 months.

Serving Size: 1 cup
Per Serving: Calories: 230; Total Fat: 1g; Total Carbs: 60g; Sugar: 45g; Fiber: 12g; Protein: 1g; Sodium: 0mg

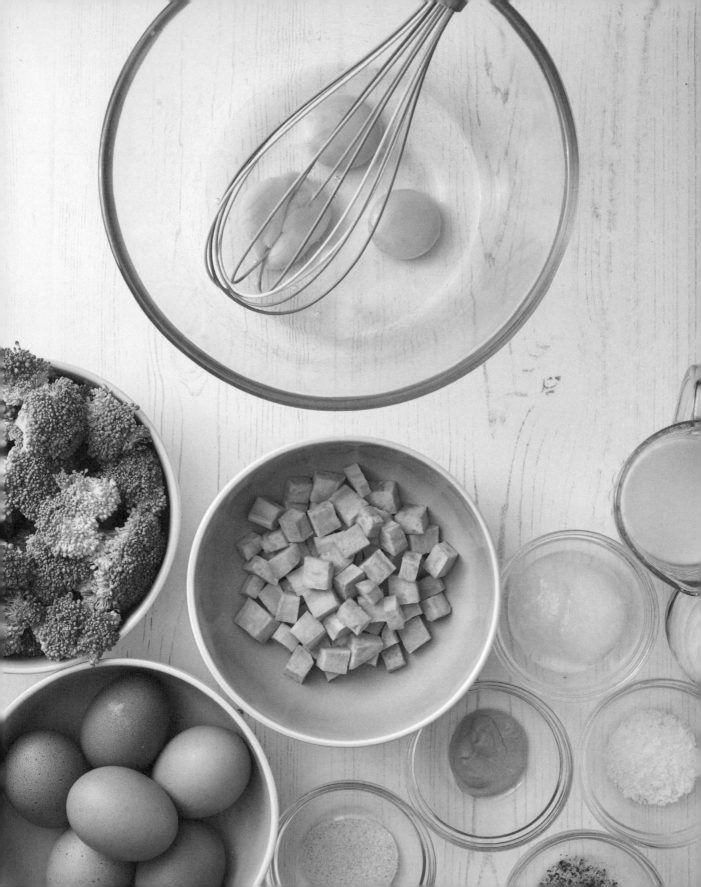

Measurement Conversions

Volume Equivalents (LIQUID)

US STANDARD	US STANDARD (OUNCES)	METRIC (APPROXIMATE)
2 tablespoons	1 fl. oz.	30 mL
¼ cup	2 fl. oz.	60 mL
½ cup	4 fl. oz.	120 mL
1 cup	8 fl. oz.	240 mL
1½ cups	12 fl. oz.	355 mL
2 cups or 1 pint	16 fl. oz.	475 mL
4 cups or 1 quart	32 fl. oz.	1 L
1 gallon	128 fl. oz.	4 L

Volume Equivalents (DRY)

US STANDARD	METRIC (APPROXIMATE)
⅛ teaspoon	0.5 mL
¼ teaspoon	1 mL
½ teaspoon	2 mL
¾ teaspoon	4 mL
1 teaspoon	5 mL
1 tablespoon	15 mL
¼ cup	59 mL
⅓ cup	79 mL
½ cup	118 mL
⅔ cup	156 mL
¾ cup	177 mL
1 cup	235 mL
2 cups or 1 pint	475 mL
3 cups	700 mL
4 cups or 1 quart	1 L

Oven Temperatures

FAHRENHEIT (F)	CELSIUS (C) (APPROXIMATE)
250°	120°
300°	150°
325°	165°
350°	180°
375°	190°
400°	200°
425°	220°
450°	230°

Weight Equivalents

US STANDARD	METRIC (APPROXIMATE)
½ ounce	15 g
1 ounce	30 g
2 ounces	60 g
4 ounces	115 g
8 ounces	225 g
12 ounces	340 g
16 ounces or 1 pound	455 g

The Dirty Dozen and the Clean Fifteen™

A nonprofit environmental watchdog organization called Environmental Working Group (EWG) looks at data supplied by the U.S. Department of Agriculture (USDA) and the Food and Drug Administration (FDA) about pesticide residues. Each year it compiles a list of the best and worst pesticide loads found in commercial crops. You can use these lists to decide which fruits and vegetables to buy organic to minimize your exposure to pesticides and which produce is considered safe enough to buy conventionally. This does not mean they are pesticide-free, though, so wash these fruits and vegetables thoroughly.

DIRTY DOZEN

apples

celery

cherries

grapes

nectarines

peaches

pears

potatoes

spinach

strawberries

sweet bell peppers

tomatoes

Additionally, nearly three-quarters of hot pepper samples contained pesticide residues

CLEAN FIFTEEN

asparagus

avocados

broccoli

cabbages

cantaloupes

cauliflower

eggplants

honeydew melons

kiwis

mangoes

onions

papayas

pineapples

sweet corn

sweet peas (frozen)

Recipe Index

Index

About the Author

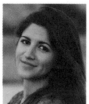 **Madeline Given** is a holistic nutritionist, author, and health educator. She works alongside women, helping them find the freedom of health in their ever-changing bodies. She is the author of *The Apple Cider Vinegar Cure* and *The Anti-Inflammatory Diet Cookbook*. For wellness wisdom and real-food ideas, visit MadelineNutrition.com or find her on Instagram and Facebook (@MadelineNutrition). She lives in Santa Barbara, California, with her husband and toddler son.